Care Support in Practice

Nessa Griffin-Heslin

BORU

PRESS

Boru Press Ltd.
The Farmyard
Birdhill
Co. Tipperary
www.borupress.ie

© Nessa Griffin-Heslin 2019

ISBN 978 19160 1992 8

Design by Sarah McCoy
Print origination by Carole Lynch
Illustrations by Andriy Yankovskyy
Printed by GraphyCems Ltd, Spain

The paper used in this book is made from wood pulp of managed forests. For every tree felled, at least one tree is planted, thereby renewing natural resources.

A CIP catalogue record for this book is available from the British Library.

For permission to reproduce photographs and artworks, the author and publisher gratefully acknowledge the following:

© Belbin 53 © Dahlgren G, Whitehead M. 33 © Department of Health 2 © HSE 2, 5, 6, 8, 173 © Dignity in Care UK 107 © Hellomynameis.org 105 © Irish Hospice Foundation 109 © Irish Workhouse Centre 2 © iStock 16, 28, 65, 93, 94, 95, 135, 165, 168 © Nessa Griffin-Heslin 64, 111 © QQI 22 © Royal College of Physicians Ireland 2 © Shutterstock 3, 19, 22, 25, 29, 30, 45, 46, 69, 72, 76, 95, 135, 143

The author and publisher have made every effort to trace all copyright holders, but if any has been inadvertently overlooked we would be pleased to make the necessary arrangement at the first opportunity.

CONTENTS

Acknowledgements

I would like to say thank you to the all providers I have had the opportunity to work with and teach this module with over the years.

Thank you to the management and staff of Longford and Westmeath Education and Training Board and Longford College of Further Education for giving me the opportunity to continue teaching this module on the Healthcare Support course.

The experiences I have had with all these people has been invaluable.

Thank you to all the students I have met over the years who have shared their experiences; their dedication to becoming carers has been inspirational and I have learned something from each and every one of them.

Thank you to Marion and Anna at Boru Press. I really appreciate their giving me the opportunity to write this book and for supporting me whilst doing so.

Thank you so much to my parents, family and friends who have listened to me about 'the book'. I am so grateful for all their support and words of wisdom.

This book is dedicated to Gary, Sam and Joel.

chapter 1

THE IRISH HEALTHCARE SYSTEM

IN THIS CHAPTER YOU WILL LEARN ABOUT:

- The history of the Irish Healthcare Service

- The structure and function of the Irish Healthcare Service today

- The differences between primary, secondary and tertiary care

- The system of charges and allowances associated with the Healthcare Service in Ireland

- The Health Information Quality Authority (HIQA)

The History of the Irish Healthcare Service

The following timeline presents an overview of some of the more important dates in the history of healthcare service in Ireland which includes the passing of key pieces of legislation upon which our current system is based. Showing these key events in their chronological order will provide an understanding of the cause and effect of those events, and allow us to step back and view the big picture of this history, of how and why events unfolded the way they did, and how these events were related.

The history of the Irish Healthcare Service is a long one dating back to 1180 with the founding of the first hospital in Dublin, the Hospital of St John the Baptist, Thomas Street. The first voluntary hospital, the Charitable Infimary, was established in Jervis Street, Dublin in 1718. The eighteenth century saw the commencement of an impoverished local authority hospital system featuring county infirmaries and fever hospitals (Hensey 1988). Voluntary hospitals were run by religious orders and philanthropic (charitable)

IRISH HEALTHCARE SERVICE TIMELINE

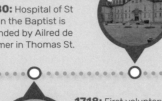

1180: Hospital of St John the Baptist is founded by Ailred de Palmer in Thomas St.

1720: Dr Steevens' Hospital, Dublin, is opened.

1747: St Patrick's Psychiatric Hospital is opened.

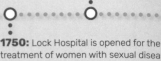

1753: Meath Hospital, Liberties, Dublin, is opened (now Tallaght Hospital).

1718: First voluntary hospital, Jervis St. Hospital (the Charitable Infirmary), is founded, followed by others in Cork, Limerick, Waterford and Belfast.

1734: Mercer Hospital, Fishamble St., is opened. Handel's Messiah is first heard here in 1742 for a hospital fundraising event.

1750: Lock Hospital is opened for the treatment of women with sexual diseases. Under the Contagious Diseases Act, women can be forcibly removed to the Lock hospitals in Dublin, the Curragh and Cork, and detained until such time as they were cured. Often they are put out of their misery, with the favourite form of euthanasia being 'smotheration' (*Irish Times* 2009).

1843: The Hospitals (Ireland) Act

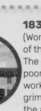

1838: The Poor Law (Workhouses) Act, The Relief of the Poor (Ireland) Act: The country is divided into poor law unions, each with a workhouse. Workhouses are grim and discourage all but the absolute destitute from partaking in their relative benefits.

1834: St Vincent's Hospital set up in St Stephen's Green, now located in Mount Merrio[n], Dublin (first Catholic hospital)

1845–52: The Great Famine – 1,000,000 deaths, 1,000,000 emigrations

1851: The Medical Charities Act – details rules and regulations regarding the dispensary service

1897: Irish Local Governme[nt] Board – recommended appointment of trained nurs[es]

2001: 'Primary Care: A New Direction; Quality and Fairness - A Health System for You' (DoHC) acknowledges the central role of primary care in the future development of the health services and proposes the introduction of an inter-disciplinary team-based approach on a phased basis using existing infrastructure and encouraging the use of public-private partnerships where practical.

1862: Poor Law (Amendment) Act – workhouse, infirmaries and fever hospitals converted into general hospitals

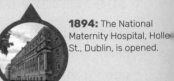

1894: The National Maternity Hospital, Holle[s] St., Dublin, is opened.

1999: The Health (ERHA) Act – establishment of the Eastern Regional Health Authority

1996: Health Amendment Act

2002: The National Primary Care Taskforce responsible for driving forward the Primary Care Strategy is established.

2000: National Health Promotion Strategy 2000–2005 is published.

An Roinn Sláinte Department of Health

1997: The Department of Health is renamed Department of Health and Children (DoHC)

2005: HSE comes into operation [on] 1 January. Health Information Qua[lity] Authority (HIQA) is established. Medical card entitlement expande[d]. New GP visit card introduced.

2003: Health Service Reform Programme – most radical structural change of the Irish Healthcare System since 1970.

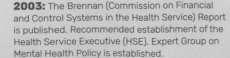

2003: The Brennan (Commission on Financial and Control Systems in the Health Service) Report is published. Recommended establishment of the Health Service Executive (HSE). Expert Group on Mental Health Policy is established.

2004: The Health Act – establishing the Health Service Executive (HSE). The Public Health (Tobacco Amendment) Act is introduced.

2007: HIQA gains full statutory status.

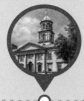

1757: The Rotunda Maternity Hospital is opened.

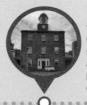

18TH AND EARLY 19TH CENTURY: The rise of infections such as tuberculosis, smallpox and typhoid fever threatens public health. This sees the establishment of fever hospitals.

1765: The County Infirmaries Act ensures the establishment of an infirmary or hospital in each Irish county.

1804: Cow-Pock Institution is set up to provide free vaccination against smallpox.

1820: Central Board of Health is established.

1818: Local Boards of Health are established.

1805: Act of Parliament – recognition of dispensaries

1829: Catholic Emancipation in Ireland

1819: Legislation enables Officers of Health to be appointed.

1810: Richmond Asylum, Grangegorman, Dublin (later known as St Brendan's Psychiatric Hospital), is opened as Ireland's first public psychiatric hospital.

1933: The Public Hospital Act

1947: The Health Act – Department of Local Government and Public Health is divided into two separate departments.

1919: Irish Public Health Council is appointed

1945: The Mental Health Treatment Act

1953: The Health Act – the role for voluntary and community organisations is recognised, permitting the government to fund voluntary organisations for health provision. Medical cards are introduced.

1957: Voluntary Health Insurance Act is passed which contributes to the developed of a two-tier health system of public and private hospital care.

1987: Health (Amendment) Act

1966: White Paper – outlines the necessity for the regionalisation of health services. There is a proposal to change GP services.

1994: 'Shaping a Healthier Future: A Strategy for Effective Health Care in the 1990s' (DoH): the first of its kind, it represented an agenda for the development of the Irish health system over a defined time period. The principles of equity, quality of service and accountability underpinned its main objective.

1994: Health (Outpatients Charges) Regulations

1970: The Health Act – eight regional Health Boards are established, covering counties in the Republic of Ireland. These health boards are divided into three areas: Community Care Services, General Hospital Services and Special Hospital Services.

2017: Launch of Sláintecare, a vision for a new health service in Ireland (see Appendix 2).

SINCE 2007, many Acts and bills passed. The Mental Health Act 2008, Nursing Home Support Scheme Act 2009 and The Protection of Life during Pregnancy Act 2013 are just three examples. For a concise list of health-related legislation, please refer to the Department of Health's website: https://health.gov.ie/publications-research/legislation/acts/

2019: Six new health regions to be developed as part of implementing Sláintecare, which will provide people with the health services they need as close to home as possible, with the majority of care delivered in the community and not in acute hospitals.

organisations and their importance grew as hospitals were transformed from providing medical relief to the poor into clinical training centres in the nineteenth century.

The eighteenth century and early nineteenth century saw the rise of infections such as tuberculosis, smallpox and typhoid fever, which threatened public health and led to the establishment of fever hospitals.

In 1805, dispensaries – institutions where medicine and advice was given freely to the poor – were legally recognised. Dispensaries did not have wards or in-patient beds and were often described as being filthy. The dispensary doctor, who often visited the sick in their homes, can be seen as a forerunner of the present-day general practitioner (GP). Supported by voluntary donations, dispensary doctors made long journeys on foot to reach their patients. They had inadequate pay and no regular pension. Many dispensary doctors died of overwork as it was a hopeless and thankless job in a system built on the necessity of bringing medical treatment to those too poor to pay for it; and like the workhouse system, its whole basis was pauperism (Geary 2004).

The Great Famine, 1845–52, brought starvation and famine-related diseases. It was responsible for more than 1,000,000 deaths in Ireland and the emigration of at least another 1,000,000.

At the time of the first potato failure in 1845, 118 workhouses were operational, some with fever hospitals attached, and the country had more than 800 medical charities, suggesting comprehensive relief and medical service for the poor. But the institutions were defective in many respects and were to prove totally inadequate in meeting the catastrophic levels of destitution, morbidity and mortality that arose during this time (Geary and HIA 2018).

The Relief of the Poor (Ireland) Act 1838, amendments in 1843 and 1847, and the 1851 Medical Charities Act were an acknowledgement of the inadequacy of philanthropy and private initiatives to deal with sickness and poverty in Ireland. The 1851 Medical Charities Act was a direct consequence of the Great

Famine. Nationwide workhouse and dispensary systems funded from rates collected from the poor were set up. These Acts represented a shift towards greater state involvement and increased centralisation (Geary and HIA 2018).

The Irish Healthcare Service Today

The Irish Healthcare System is a two-tier system consisting of both private and public sectors. The private sector means that people can have private health insurance and pay for care and be attended to in private clinics and hospitals, which usually have shorter waiting times for appointments and treatment. The public sector is run by the Health Service Executive (HSE) and is funded by general taxation. Everyone resident in Ireland is entitled to receive healthcare through the public healthcare system.

The current healthcare system in Ireland is governed by the Health Act 2004. On 1 January 2005, the HSE was established under this Act. The HSE replaced the previous system, which was made up of ten regional Health Boards, the Eastern Regional Health Authority and various other agencies and organisations.

HSE Divisions

Up to 2019 the HSE was divided into four administrative regions: Dublin North East, Dublin Mid Leinster, South and West. It delivered a range of services through 50 hospitals and 32 health offices nationally (See Appendix 1 HSE 4 Administrative Areas and 50 Acute Care Hospitals).

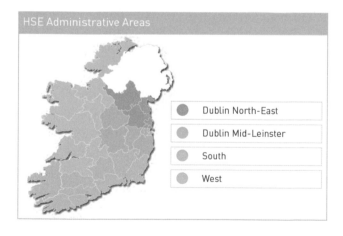

HSE Administrative Areas

- Dublin North-East
- Dublin Mid-Leinster
- South
- West

Since 2004 there has been no major changes to the structure of the HSE. In 2019, significant changes featuring the introduction of six new health regions for Ireland were announced by the government. These will replace the current structure of the HSE.

The establishment of new regions is part of Sláintecare, the ten-year blueprint for the reform of the health service introduced in 2017. The aim is to deliver health services to people as close to their homes as possible with the majority of care delivered in the community and not in acute hospitals (See Appendix 2 Sláintecare- A Pathway to Universal Healthcare in Ireland).

For more information about the changes, refer to the HSE website (www.hse.ie). For more information about Sláintecare Implementation Strategy, refer to www.gov.ie.

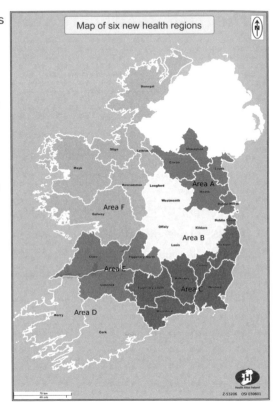

Map of six new health regions

The HSE's vision is to have 'a healthier Ireland with a high-quality health service valued by all'. Its core values are care, compassion, trust and learning. Its mission is to ensure that people in Ireland:

+ are supported by health and social care services to achieve their full potential

+ can access safe, compassionate and quality care when they need it

+ can be confident that the HSE will deliver the best outcomes and value through optimising their resources.

(HSE 2015)

The HSE takes responsibility for the delivery of all publicly funded health and social services nationally. It is responsible for the following services to the public (HSE, 2018):

Publicly Funded Health and Social Services

+ Acute hospitals

+ Social care

+ Mental health

+ Primary care

+ Health and wellbeing

+ National Ambulance Service

HSE Community Healthcare Services

The HSE also provides community healthcare services outside of the acute hospital system, such as primary care, social care, mental health plus health and wellbeing services. Each county in the Republic of Ireland is covered by a community health service.

+ **Area 1:** Cavan, Donegal, Leitrim, Monaghan, Sligo

+ **Area 2:** Community Healthcare West

+ **Area 3:** Mid-West Community Healthcare

+ **Area 4:** Cork Kerry Community Healthcare

+ **Area 5:** South East Community Healthcare

+ **Area 6:** Community Healthcare East

+ **Area 7:** Dublin South/Dublin West/Dublin South-West/Kildare and West Wicklow Community Healthcare

+ **Area 8:** Midlands: Louth, Meath, Longford, Westmeath Community Healthcare

+ **Area 9:** Dublin North City and County Community Healthcare

HSE Other Services

The HSE provides thousands of services to people of all ages in hospitals, health centres and communities. Some of these services include:

+ Hospital services

+ Public nursing services

+ Child health services

+ Occupational therapy

+ Addiction counselling

+ GP services

+ Social work

+ Home help

+ Speech therapy

The Structure of the Health Service Executive (HSE)

The service is provided in three areas of care known as:

Feidhmeannacht na Seirbhíse Sláinte
Health Service Executive

1. Primary

2. Secondary

3. Tertiary.

Primary Care

Primary care is the first point of contact that people have with health and social service needs i.e. through GP or public health nurses. It is provided in primary care settings such as GP surgeries or health offices within the local community. It is delivered by a primary care team, outside of the hospital setting, and can include a range of services from health screening to assessment, diagnosis, rehabilitation and care in the home (HSE

2018a). The primary care team is responsible for organising and delivering primary healthcare for the local population and can consist of GPs, nurses, physiotherapists, speech and language therapists and occupational therapists. The aim of the primary care team is to provide accessible, integrated, high-quality services to meet the needs of the local population. They provide clients with a single point of contact to the healthcare system.

The following is a list of members of the primary healthcare team:

+ General practitioners (GPs)
+ Practice nurse services
+ Community pharmacists
+ Dieticians
+ Community welfare officers
+ Dentists
+ Chiropodists/podiatrists
+ Psychologists/counselling

+ Home help/health care assistant (HCA) services
+ Physiotherapists
+ Occupational therapists
+ Social workers
+ Administration personnel
+ Speech and language therapists

Task **Stop and think!**

Can you think of a primary care centre in your locality?

What services are available there?

Is it easy to access?

Secondary Care

Secondary care is provided in an acute hospital setting. This is necessary for seriously ill and injured clients or those requiring further tests, diagnosis and treatment. Some clients are admitted following an accident, injury or sudden illness while some are referred by their GP. Other clients self-refer.

Members of the secondary healthcare team include:

+ Consultants
+ Nurses
+ HCAs
+ Advanced nurse practitioner
+ Clinical nurse specialists
+ Porters
+ Catering staff
+ Occupational therapists
+ Physiotherapists
+ Social workers
+ Psychologists
+ Speech and language therapists
+ Dieticians
+ Administration staff
+ Educators
+ Student nurses/midwives/ doctors
+ Chaplain
+ Resuscitation officers.

Tertiary Care

Tertiary care is specialised consultative care, usually on referral from primary or secondary care team members. It is provided in cases where a client requires a higher level of specialty investigation, treatment and care e.g. severe burns, renal dialysis, brain surgery. It is normally confined to a small number of locations which have specialised equipment and personnel with specialised expertise (DOHC 2001).

Charges for Healthcare Services

Ireland has a comprehensive, government-funded public healthcare system. A person living in Ireland for at least one year is considered by the HSE to be 'ordinarily resident' and is entitled to either full eligibility (Category 1) or limited eligibility (Category 2) for health services.

Category 1

People with medical cards can access a wide range of health services and medicines free of charge. They are entitled to the following:

+ Free hospital care

+ GP visits

+ Dental services

+ Optical services

+ Aural services

+ Some prescription drugs

+ Medical appliances

Medical card eligibility is based on an individual's income, expenses, marital status and dependants.

Category 2

People without medical cards can access a wide range of community and hospital health services, either free of charge or at a reduced cost. Maternity services, child medical care up to the age of six months and long-term illness care are free. Under the Drugs Payment Scheme (DPS), an individual or family will pay no more than €124 each calendar month for approved prescribed drugs and medicines or rental costs for respiratory equipment.

General Practitioner visit cards may be awarded to those on a slightly higher income which entitles the holder to free general practitioner visits. General Practitioner visit cards are available to carers in receipt of carer's benefit or carer's allowance, adults over 70 years of age and children up to the age of six. Those not qualifying for either medical cards or GP visit cards must pay for GP visits at a rate set by the GP.

There are several types of hospital charges, which include:

+ Emergency department charges; without being referred by your GP or family doctor, the charge is €100. There is no charge if you are referred (with a letter) by your GP.

+ Out-patient charges (same as emergency department charges)

+ Daily in-patient charges (€80 per day)

+ Long-term stay charges (maximum of €175 per week).

(Citizens Information, 2019 and HSE, 2018)

The Health Information Quality Authority (HIQA)

The Health Information Quality Authority (HIQA) was established under the Health Act 2007. It is an independent body which reports to the Minister for Health and works closely with the Minister for Children and Youth Affairs.

HIQA's role is to:

+ develop standards

+ inspect health and social care facilities.

in order to promote quality and safety for the benefit of the health and welfare of the public (www.HIQA.ie).

HIQA Standards

+ National Standards for Children's Residential Centres – 7 November 2018

+ National Standards for Infection Prevention and Control in Community Services – 19 September 2018

+ Background Document to Support the Development of National Standards for Adult Safeguarding – 9 May 2018

+ National Standards for the Conduct of Reviews of Patient Safety Incidents – 25 October 2017

+ National Standards for the Prevention and Control of Healthcare-Associated Infections in Acute Healthcare Services – 23 May 2017

+ National Standards for Safer Better Maternity Services – 21 December 2016

+ Current: National Standards for Residential Care Settings for Older People in Ireland – 3 May 2016

+ National Standards for Special Care Units – 3 March 2015

+ National Standards for Residential Services for Children and Adults with Disabilities – 14 May 2013

+ National Standards for the Protection and Welfare of Children – 25 July 2012

+ National Standards for Safer Better Healthcare – 26 June 2012

+ Previous: National Standards for the Prevention and Control of Healthcare Associated Infections – 27 May 2009

+ Previous: National Quality Standards for Residential Care Settings for Older People in Ireland – 9 March 2009

+ Previous: Quality Assurance Standards for Symptomatic Breast Disease Services in Ireland – 18 February 2007

Further standards and information about publications can be found on the HIQA website https://www.hiqa.ie/reports-and-publications/standards

HIQA Inspections

HIQA carry out inspections of healthcare and social services to monitor and protect vulnerable clients by ensuring that service providers are complying with legislation and national standards. HIQA can require changes to be made in line with recommendations from previous inspections to ensure the best quality of care. HIQA will also carry out an inspection if there has been a complaint about a service provider. These are the following inspection processes:

+ **Registration inspection:** Carried out when a service has applied to register or re-register a centre.

+ **Announced inspection:** The centre will be aware of the inspection dates.

✦ **Unannounced inspection:** The centre will be unaware of this inspection until the inspectors turn up at the door.

> ## HIQA Areas of Work:
>
> ✦ Acute and community healthcare services
>
> ✦ Children's services
>
> ✦ Disability services
>
> ✦ Older people's services
>
> ✦ Health information
>
> ✦ Health technology assessment
>
> ✦ HRB-CICER clinical guideline support (The Health Research Board – Collaboration in Ireland for Clinical Effectiveness Reviews)
>
> ✦ Standards and quality
>
> *Source:* https://www.hiqa.ie/

Relevance of HIQA to the HCA

Why Is It Important for HCAs to Know about HIQA?
Prior to a Job Interview

At a job interview it is very likely that the HCA will be asked to communicate what they know about HIQA, its aims, role and what it does. Prior to an interview, the HCA should refresh all knowledge of HIQA, especially their published standards for the area in which the HCA hopes to work; for example, if the HCA is interviewing for work in an elderly people's facility, knowledge of the National Quality Standards for Residential Care Settings for Older People in Ireland (2016) will be essential.

In the Workplace

Once employed, the HCA must be aware of and clearly understand the specific workplace policies and procedures, particularly the Statement of

Purpose as clearly identified in Theme 5 Standard 5.3 of the HIQA Standards. The HCA should also know and clearly understand the standards as they apply to the quality of care for the clients being looked after in addition to the policies and procedures specific to the place of work. The HCA needs knowledge and awareness of:

+ Infection control

+ Individual choice (relating to food, clothing and social activities) for residents

+ Dignity, privacy and independence

+ Safeguarding of clients and promoting a care environment free from restrictive practices (HIQA 2019)

+ Standards of care

+ Legislation

+ Safety and health at work e.g. fall prevention, fire, moving and handling

+ Pressure area care

+ Managing behaviours that challenge e.g. Management of Actual or Potential Aggression (MAPA)

+ Dementia care.

There may be other specific areas for which the HCA may be required to undergo special training. The manager/supervisor should be able to advise and, when necessary and appropriate, arrange training.

chapter 2

ROLE OF THE HEALTH CARE ASSISTANT

IN THIS CHAPTER YOU WILL LEARN ABOUT:

- The role of the Health Care Assistant (HCA)
- History and development of the HCA role
- Responsibilities and tasks of the HCA
- Qualities and characteristics required
- Opportunities for career progression

The Role of the HCA

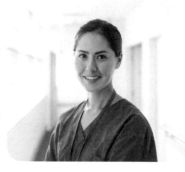

The role of the Health Care Assistant (HCA) is to deliver client care under the direction and supervision of the registered nurse/midwife/public health nurse as appropriate (DOHC 2001).

HCAs can also be referred to as:

- Health care attendants
- Carers
- Care assistants
- Nursing assistants
- Nurse's aides
- Ward orderlies
- Support workers.

In Ireland these are generally known as HCAs.

History and Development of the HCA Role

The role of the HCA has changed over time. It was previously a position for which formal education and training was not required. Hospitals and care facilities did provide in-house education that was beneficial; however, this in-house training was not accredited by a national body. The training had to include certain aspects such as patient moving and handling, and fire training (Duffy 2008).

Over time it was recognised that the roles of nurses, midwives and HCAs were changing and expanding. The *Report on the Commission on Nursing, A Blueprint for the Future* (DOHC 1998) recommended the development of the HCA role in order to help with the increasing responsibilities of the nurse/midwife. It was deemed necessary that to develop the function of the HCA, they needed to be educated to a certain standard to ensure they were competent and safe practitioners. This was highlighted in *Effective Utilisation of Professional Skills of Nurses and Midwives Report of the Working Group* (DOHC 2001).

The report recommended that HCAs be educated to a Level 2 qualification under the National Council for Vocational Awards (NCVA). Shortly after, this was changed to a Further Education and Training Awards Council (FETAC) award and is currently a Quality and Qualification Ireland (QQI) award.

The programme was piloted in numerous locations in 2001 and was very successful. All HCAs must now be educated to QQI Level 5 in order to work in healthcare settings. There are numerous QQI Level 5 healthcare courses available including:

+ QQI Level 5 Healthcare Support Course 5M4339

+ QQI Level 5 Health Service Skills 5M3782

+ QQI Level 5 Community Care 5M2786

+ QQI Level 5 Nursing Studies 5M4349.

The role of the HCA will depend on the place of work. The HCA should be aware of their job description so that they know and clearly understand what they are, and are not, expected to do. The HCA is expected to understand the needs of the client, to treat them with dignity and respect always. Their role is to assist the nurse in implementing care to the client. The HCA works within a Multidisciplinary Team (MDT), under the guidance and supervision of the nurse/midwife.

The *Effective Utilisation of Professional Skills of Nurses and Midwives Report of the Working Group* (DOHC 2001) outlines a national job description for HCAs (see Appendix 3).

> **Task** **Stop and think!**
> Spend a few moments thinking about all the jobs a HCA might be required to do.

Responsibilities and Tasks of the HCA

In general, the role of the HCA includes assisting clients with some or all the Activities of Daily Living (ADLs) (see page 117) along with other tasks including the following:

+ **Personal care:** Washing and dressing, bathing, showering, combing hair, shaving, checking fingernails/toenails, foot care

+ **Pressure area care:** Observing, reporting

+ **Performing observations:** Blood pressures, temperatures, pulses, respirations, oxygen saturations

+ **Mobility:** Assisting with walking, using equipment, wheelchairs, rollators, walking sticks, hoists

+ **Eating and drinking:** Assisting with eating and drinking, serving food and drink, being aware of modified diets, people with differing needs e.g. dysphagia, diabetes

+ **Elimination needs:** Assisting client to the toilet, changing continence wear, changing stoma bags, emptying catheter bags

+ **Communication:** Assisting in communication with family, clients and other staff members

- **Documentation and record-keeping:** Reporting changes in client's condition, filling out documents as per workplace policy

- **Maintaining client safety:** Prevention of falls, removal of obstacles, lighting, fire safety

- **Safeguarding of clients:** Monitoring for signs of abuse

- **Infection control prevention:** Standard precautions, handwashing, disposal of linen, disposal of waste, cleaning, isolation procedures, personal protective equipment, uniforms, personal wellness

- **Maintaining a clean environment:** Cleaning equipment

- **Reporting broken equipment:** As stated in the written policy of the home or hospital in which the HCA is working

- **Stocktaking:** Checking the stock on the ward, department or nursing home for e.g. linen, waste bags, aprons, gloves, continence wear etc. to ensure staff and clients are never short of necessary equipment.

The HCA can work in public and private healthcare sectors in different areas:

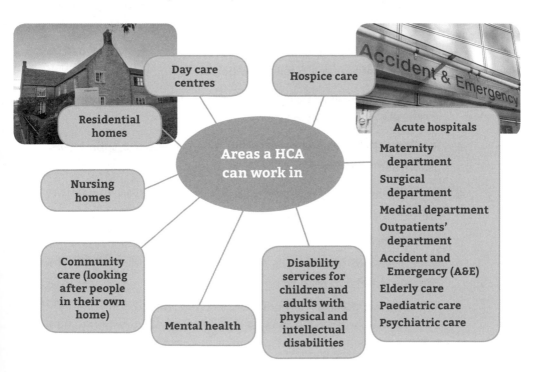

Qualities and Characteristics Required of the HCA

The HCA will be given jobs by the nurse/midwife, but must **never** do anything that they do not feel competent or safe to do. If there are any doubts, tell the supervisor/person in charge, who will offer help and guidance.

As well as having different jobs to carry out whilst at work, the HCA needs to have a good work ethic. This means taking pride in being a HCA and doing all jobs to the very best of their ability. In order to do this, there are various qualities/characteristics required:

+ **Professionalism:** Being punctual for the shift, having a clean, tidy presentation, wearing a uniform and name badge, speaking to people in the correct tone and manner by being courteous and respectful

+ **Reliability:** Being available, flexible

+ **Accountability:** Taking responsibility for own work, not doing jobs you are not trained to do, lack competency in or feel unsure/unsafe to do without guidance or support from the nurse or supervisor

+ **Empathy:** Seeing things from other people's perspectives whether they be clients or their family members

+ **Conscientiousness:** Being hardworking, dedicated to care work and to the centre you are in

+ **Honesty:** Being honest with other team members, supervisors, clients and family members

+ **Desire to learn:** Being willing to learn and develop skills. Continuing Professional Development (CPD) is vital for good quality care and standards.

+ **Good sense of humour:** Having a good attitude. Working in care can be stressful and tiring and dealing with emotional and sometimes fraught situations can leave us feeling worn-out and sometimes downhearted. Having a good sense of humour can help to lift that mood, provided it is used at the right times!

+ **Good communication skills:** Listening, handing over important information about clients that could potentially save their life

+ **Good team player:** Working with other people, listening to their opinions, knowing when to ask for help

+ **Treating people with dignity and respect:** Remembering they are human beings with feelings

+ **Maintaining confidentiality:** Never passing information on to anyone about a client who doesn't need to know about their care requirements.

(Power 2019, Carter and Goldschmidt, 2010)

Opportunities for Career Progression

Upon completion of any of the QQI Level 5 healthcare courses, there are many opportunities for career development and progression.

Employment

A qualified HCA can gain employment in both the public and private sector. Within the HSE job opportunities can be obtained in acute hospitals, hospices, private and public nursing homes, residential homes, home care agencies, residential care for children and adults with intellectual disabilities, maternity and children's hospitals and mental health services.

Continuing Education

A HCA can progress in education to the following courses:

+ QQI Level 6 Health Service Supervisory Management Skills 6M4978
+ QQI Level 6 Community Development 6M3674.

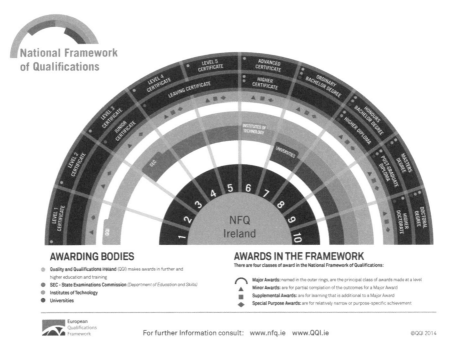

National Framework of Qualifications

AWARDING BODIES

● Quality and Qualifications Ireland (QQI) makes awards in further and higher education and training
● SEC - State Examinations Commission (Department of Education and Skills)
● Institutes of Technology
● Universities

AWARDS IN THE FRAMEWORK

There are four classes of award in the National Framework of Qualifications:

⌒ **Major Awards:** named in the outer rings, are the principal class of awards made at a level
▲ **Minor Awards:** are for partial completion of the outcomes for a Major Award
■ **Supplemental Awards:** are for learning that is additional to a Major Award
◆ **Special Purpose Awards:** are for relatively narrow or purpose-specific achievement

European Qualifications Framework

For further Information consult: www.nfq.ie   www.QQI.ie

©QQI 2014

There are options to continue education within the fields of nursing or midwifery within the institutes of technology or colleges in the UK or Scotland. An applied social studies course is another option for progression, offered at a variety of educational institutions in Ireland.

If further education is part of the HCA's overall career plan, it is vital that they choose the most appropriate and relevant modules at Level 5 in order to ensure successful application to higher-level courses. Discuss this with the career advisor or healthcare course tutor/co-ordinator.

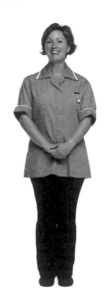

The role of the HCA is always evolving so Continuing Professional Development (CPD) is important, particularly in the areas of:

✚ Infection prevention and control including hand hygiene

✚ Pressure area care

✚ Safeguarding vulnerable people

✚ Responding to challenging behaviour

✚ Manual handling

✚ Cardiopulmonary Resuscitation (CPR)

✚ National Early Warning Score (NEWS) in an acute hospital

✚ Dementia care

✚ Trust in care

✚ Dignity at work.

Other areas will be relevant to your place of work or whatever your employer recommends.

(HSE.ie)

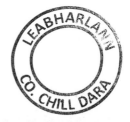

chapter 3

WORKING IN DIFFERENT CARE ENVIRONMENTS

IN THIS CHAPTER YOU WILL LEARN ABOUT:

+ Various working environments for Health Care Assistants (HCAs)

+ How each environment differs from others

+ Services each care environment offers and how they suit different clients

The specific job description of a healthcare worker depends on the healthcare facility in which they work. We will examine the main providers of job opportunities for HCAs as follows:

+ Hospitals

+ Nursing homes

+ Home care environments

+ Other care environments

Working in Hospitals

In Ireland there are both public and private hospitals. HCAs can work in both. Hospitals are busy places made up of wards, departments and offices working together to provide the care necessary for the client. Clients will be of all ages, presenting with various care needs on a 24/7 basis. Most hospitals will provide the following services:

- Accident and Emergency (A&E)
- Cardiac care services
- Medical care services
- Stroke services
- Surgical wards
- Maternity care
- Paediatric care
- Mental health services
- Outpatient clinics for various appointments
- Radiology, magnetic resonance imaging (MRI), X-ray
- Physiotherapy
- Occupational therapy
- Dietetics
- Speech and language therapy
- End-of-life care
- Endoscopy units
- Social work
- Rheumatology.

The more specialised hospitals will have units for brain injuries, renal (kidney) disease, burns, cancer care, maxillofacial care and sexual health.

Within the hospital you will find many members of the Multidisciplinary Team (MDT) (see Chapter 6) such as:

- advanced nurse practitioners for many areas
- administration staff
- clinical nurse specialists for many areas
- consultants for all specialities
- dieticians
- doctors for all areas
- HCAs
- housekeeping staff
- midwives
- nurses in all departments
- occupational therapists

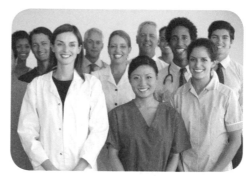

+ oncologists

+ pharmacists

+ phlebotomists (people who take blood)

+ physiotherapists

+ porters

+ social workers

+ speech and language therapists.

Depending on where you work in the hospital you may look after people with a variety of conditions. These clients may be acutely unwell, meaning they will need immediate attention and treatment from the MDT. This can be challenging. The HCA will need to be attentive, quick-thinking and able to take direction from the team.

General Conditions of Working in a Hospital

+ The turnover of clients will be much quicker in a hospital setting than in a residential facility – the HCA may not get to meet the clients' family members.

+ Depending on the department, the HCA will more than likely be expected to do shift work.

+ A uniform and name badge must be worn to identify the HCA.

+ The HCA will need to continue with their professional development and keep up to date with training in areas such as:

  – infection control

  – patient moving and handling

  – safeguarding vulnerable adults at risk of abuse (HSE 2014)

  – basic life support

  – heartsaver CPR

  – National Early Warning Score (NEWS)

  – Management of Actual and Potential Aggression (MAPA).

Working in Nursing Homes

There are public and private nursing homes in Ireland that HCAs can choose to work in. Nursing homes can vary in size with some offering only 30–40 beds or fewer, while others may have over 100. It is common today for nursing homes to also have specialist dementia or Alzheimer units.

Reasons for admittance to nursing homes include:

+ long-term illness care progressing to palliative care
+ dependency care
+ social inclusion
+ respite care
+ palliative care.

Nursing homes are usually an option for clients who are elderly, although sometimes younger clients are admitted if there are no available beds in other facilities. Nursing home residencies can often be long term with clients having varying dependency needs from low to high, meaning some will require limited help and some will require full nursing care.

Nursing homes also offer care for those who are no longer able to care for themselves or live independently, or are an option for people who *can* live independently but who feel afraid in their own homes and wish to be in a safe and secure environment – these are called social admissions.

Nursing homes are frequently used for respite purposes, with clients admitted for a short period of time – one or two weeks – usually following surgical treatment in an acute hospital.

General Conditions of Working in a Nursing Home

+ Be aware that employment within a nursing home is likely to involve shift work (day and night shifts) as well as weekend and bank holiday work.
+ A uniform and badge is mandatory.

✛   A HCA is required to have a Level 5 award in a healthcare subject to gain employment and will be expected to continue professional development in areas including:

-   Health Information Quality Authority (HIQA) regulations

-   infection control (handwashing)

-   patient moving and handling

-   safeguarding vulnerable adults at risk of abuse (HSE 2014)

-   basic life support

-   fire training

-   dementia care.

Working in Home Care

There are numerous home care agencies in Ireland that a HCA could work for. Home care agencies employ HCAs to visit clients in their homes on appointed days and times. The type of care required, and the frequency of the visits, are determined by the public health nurse and based on an 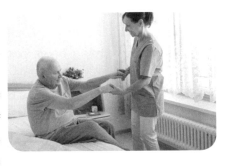 assessment of the client's needs. The clients could be of varying ages and present with varying conditions and needs such as:

✛   dementia

✛   cerebral palsy

✛   general ageing conditions

✛   stroke conditions

✛   Multiple Sclerosis (MS)

✛   motor neurone disease

✛   palliative care

✛   people who have had accidents.

Some clients will have social needs, such as requiring help with preparing meals, or may only require a minimal amount of help with washing and dressing. At the other end of the scale there will be those who have higher dependency needs and will require full and total care. The HCA may work alone, although some clients may require two carers.

General Conditions of Working in Home Care

✚ Being able to drive is an advantage as you will be assigned clients in different locations. However, it may be possible for you to walk, cycle or use public transport to travel to visit your clients depending on the circumstances and the policy of the home care agency.

✚ Good organisational skills and time management is important so you can get to your visits within the time allocated and not leave your client waiting for you.

✚ You may need a uniform (depending on the policy of the agency) and will be required to have a form of identification.

✚ It will be necessary to continue with your professional development and keep up to date with training such as Infection Control, Patient Moving and Handling, Safeguarding Vulnerable Adults at Risk of Abuse (HSE, 2014).

Working in Other Care Environments

There are many other care environments that you could choose to work in.

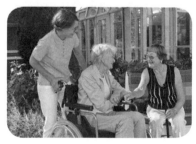

✚ **Hospices:** Provide care for clients who are dying, as well as support for their families. They also care for people who need respite or symptom control e.g. pain control. There are nine in-patient hospices in Ireland: three in the Dublin area and one each in Cork, Limerick, Galway, Sligo, Donegal and Kildare (https://hospicefoundation.ie/about-hospice-care/hospice-services-in-ireland/). Most palliative care is delivered in the form of home care, although acute hospitals have palliative care services too. There are some hospice/palliative care beds available in specialist units and nursing homes. The focus of hospice care is the provision of comfort and care in a holistic person-centred approach. This means looking after the client's physical, social, spiritual and psychological wellbeing and also involves looking after the client's family. Working in a hospice as a HCA, you will work as part of a large multidisciplinary team to meet the many and varied needs of the client and members of their family. To work in the area of palliative care, completing the QQI Level 5 Palliative Care Support Module 5N3769 would be beneficial.

✚ **Day Centres and Day Care Centres:** Offer social and rehabilitative services for older people and people with disabilities, and generally open during weekdays and regular working hours. These services can include chiropody, grooming 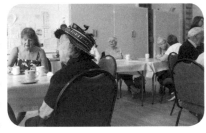 and bathing, laundry services, social and recreational activities as well as providing nutritional meals. Most day centres are provided directly by the HSE while others are provided in conjunction with voluntary organisations (https://www.citizensinformation.ie/en/).

✚ **Intellectual Disability Units:** Offer day care facilities, respite or long-stay services. Here, HCAs work with clients of all different ages with a range of intellectual and emotional disabilities.

General Conditions of Working In Other Care Environments

Each establishment will have its own mission statement, rules and regulations that HCAs must be aware of and clearly understand. Most types of care organisations require staff to wear a uniform, but a few do not. Shift work is an expected feature of care work, as care is required on a 24/7 basis, but employment is available within some centres on a part-time basis and for a regular Monday–Friday working week.

Remember

✚ Working in all these care environments can be emotionally and physically draining, however, as with all care work, it can be exceptionally rewarding. You will be helping people when they are at their most vulnerable and you can make a huge difference to their lives and to those of their loved ones. Every day will be different and you will need to be flexible and ready to meet any challenges that this variety brings.

✚ Remember, you must make your supervisor aware of any problems/issues you may have at any time. Keep up to date with current education and go on courses when recommended or requested, which will improve your knowledge, ability and self-confidence in the area in which you work.

chapter 4

HEALTH PROMOTION IN THE CARE SETTING

IN THIS CHAPTER YOU WILL LEARN ABOUT:

+ Health promotion

+ The issues and conditions that determine and affect health

+ Factors that influence and determine health

+ How to promote health in three different care settings

What Is Health Promotion?

Before we talk about the meaning of health promotion, it is important to talk about health and being healthy. The concept of health is complex and can mean different things to different people. Health has been defined as:

> A resource for everyday life, not the objective of living, making it a positive concept, emphasising social and personal resources as well as physical capabilities.
>
> (WHO 1986)

This means that we need social and personal resources as well as physical functioning in order to attain and retain good health.

Task **Stop and think!**
What does being healthy mean to you?

Being healthy can be described in many ways; 'being able to achieve one's full potential' could be one of the them (Benson 2000). Being healthy can be viewed from a holistic viewpoint where we look at the physical, psychological, spiritual and social wellbeing of a person.

The concept of health and being healthy is open to interpretation, resulting in many conflicting perspectives. If you consider that the practice of taking medication may reflect an unhealthy image, does that hold true for the young woman on long-term medication for epilepsy? There are many factors that can influence and determine health, some leading to many problems and development of diseases. These are identified in the Dahlgren-Whitehead Rainbow model of health (1992).

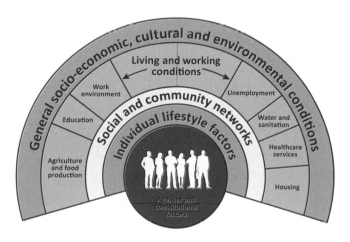

Dahlgren G, Whitehead M. (1991). *Policies and Strategies to Promote Social Equity in Health*. Stockholm, Sweden: Institute for Futures Studies

This model illustrates how health issues can be determined by social, economic and environmental factors. At an individual level, factors such as age, sex, hereditary and lifestyle choices are also important. This was identified in the *National Health Promotion Strategy 2000–2005* (DOHC 2000). Taking these factors into account, we can identify various lifestyle choices and recognise the importance of health promotion.

Health promotion is the action taken to encourage or help people to maintain or improve their health and general wellbeing. Health promotion is central to the prevention of ill health, the maintenance of health and the recognition of optimum health and wellbeing (Elcock 2019). The HSE in its Health Promotion Strategic Framework (HPSF) 2011 advocates that the overall goal of health promotion is to 'enhance positive health and prevent ill health' (HSE 2011) by addressing the broad determinants of health and health inequalities, through health services, community and education settings.

World Health Organization (WHO) Principles of Health Promotion

1. Empowerment health promotion initiatives should enable individuals and communities to assume more power over the personal, socio-economic and environmental factors that affect their health.

2. Participative health promotion initiatives should involve those concerned in all stages of planning, implementation and evaluation.

3. Holistic health promotion initiatives should foster physical, mental, social and spiritual health.

4. Inter-sectoral health promotion initiatives should involve the collaboration of agencies from relevant sectors.

5. Equitable health promotion initiatives should be guided by a concern for equity and social justice.

6. Sustainable health promotion initiatives should bring about changes that individuals and communities can maintain once initial funding has ended.

7. Multi-strategy health promotion initiatives should use a variety of approaches in combination with one another, including: policy development, organisational change, community development, legislation, advocacy, education and communication.

(Rootman 2001)

Importance of Health Promotion

Task Stop and think!
What is the importance of health promotion?

Aims and Benefits of Health Promotion

Health promotion:

+ Improves the health status of individuals, families, communities, countries and the nation

+ Enhances the quality of life for people and increases life expectancy

+ Reduces the costs to healthcare

+ Reduces health inequalities

+ Promotes healthy lifestyles by education about disorders and potential health problems

+ Promotes health screening as a preventative tool to detect disease for early treatment

+ Is not just carried out in healthcare settings, but in many other settings including schools, workplaces and youth facilities in order to reach the widest possible audience.

+ Involves three key settings: the health service, the community, education settings

(HSE 2011)

Health Promotion for the Individual

On an individual level, health promotion can be important for the following reasons:

+ It contributes to an overall sense of wellbeing including physical, psychological, social and spiritual aspects.

+ It encourages the individual to attend screening processes e.g. breast check, cervical check, prostate, so that early identification of health-related problems can be detected.

+ It brings awareness to the individual about the improvement of body function e.g. mobility.

+ It highlights positive feelings that come with good health which can reduce feelings of low mood/depression.

+ It can suggest diet changes and exercise regimes to help with weight loss and improve overall fitness.

Task

Stop and think!
Think of ways healthcare professionals can promote health in different care settings e.g. hospital, home care and hursing home.

Case Study: **David**

David is a 50-year-old man who has been admitted to the ward on which you work with a chest infection. He is Short of Breath (SOB) on arrival and requires oxygen at times. David is a very big man, overweight and struggles to walk due to the SOB and the chest infection. He spends most of his time in bed. One morning whilst you are helping him wash, he mentions, 'I'm absolutely dying for a cigarette. I can't wait till I feel better so I can go outside and have one.'

1. What would your response be to this statement?

2. Do you think there is an opportunity for you to engage in health promotion activities here?

3. Do you think David would listen?

4. Are there any other areas of David's life that may need addressing from a health promotion point of view?

Considerations for this Case Study

This may be a perfect opportunity for a discussion with David as you are with him on a one-to-one basis in a private setting. However, we must be very careful not to offend or dictate to a person. As healthcare professionals, we can only make suggestions. The person must be ready and prepared to make the changes in their current lifestyle which may be adversely affecting their health. If they are not both ready and strongly motivated, any changes they do make may be short lived and they are likely to fall back into their unhealthy ways and habits. David has not expressed a desire to stop smoking. On the contrary, he has a strong desire to have a cigarette despite being in hospital with a severe chest infection. On discharge the nurse will be able to advise David and give some information to him about stopping smoking and the support available to him.

Another area of David's life that requires addressing would be his weight. Again, this would need to be handled very sensitively. David could be referred by the nurse to a dietician for them to discuss a weight-loss plan. Your role would be to report information back to David's key nurse for them to make the relevant assessment to change the care plan.

How Can We Promote Health in Care Settings?

Promotion of health in care settings is very individualised. There are many different diseases, disabilities and conditions. Each person you come across will have a different attitude. Some will be ready to change, and others may not recognise or accept that a change is essential to regain good health and full fitness. You may work in a nursing home where you will meet 80-year-olds who smoke and who tell you that they will 'never give up'.

The table below gives a few suggestions of how health can be promoted in three different healthcare settings.

Nursing Homes	Home Care	Hospitals
Health education classes conducted by a pharmacist or other expert	Exercises	Exercises (depending on the ward/unit) Physiotherapy
Exercise classes	Monitoring of weight	Monitoring of weight
Physiotherapy	Social activities/ outings	Visits by family and friends
Monitoring of weight	Choice of food	Choice of food
Social activities/ outings	Health screening and medical check-ups – blood pressure, routine bloods, cholesterol, blood sugar, hearing, eyes, dental	Education with leaflets, referral to appropriate multidisciplinary team members e.g. dietician, speech and language therapist, occupational therapist
Choice of food	Encourage mobility	Encourage independence
Health screening and medical check-ups – blood pressure, routine bloods, cholesterol, blood sugar, hearing, eyes, dental	Promote good hygiene to prevent infection	Infection control procedures throughout hospital
Encouraging independence	Observe living conditions e.g. damp, mould, out-of-date food	Safety procedures e.g. fire regulations
Infection control procedures	Safety procedures – accidents, smoke detector	No smoking policies
Safety procedures e.g. fire regulations	Encourage no smoking	Alcohol policies

Nursing Homes	Home Care	Hospitals
No smoking policies	Education re: alcohol consumption	Education re: medications and side effects
Education re: alcohol consumption	Education re: medications and side effects	Education re: illegal drugs
Education re: medications and side effects		

Source: DOHC 2000; Nifast 2013.

chapter 5

EMPLOYMENT LEGISLATION AND INFORMATION

IN THIS CHAPTER YOU WILL LEARN ABOUT:

+ Relevant and current employment legislation

+ Employee entitlements

It is important for anyone working in care support to be aware that there are employment laws in Ireland that protect the rights of employees in the workplace. By familiarising yourself with the basic legislation and knowing where to access the information, you will be well equipped for the working world. The Department of Business, Enterprise and Innovation (DBEI) is responsible for implementing and developing government policy and for protecting the working conditions of employees.

Employment Legislation

The current employment legislation relevant to employees in Ireland are as follows:

+ **Redundancy Payments Acts 1967–2014:** Provide for a minimum entitlement to a redundancy payment for employees who have a set period of service with the employer when made redundant. Not all employees are entitled to the statutory redundancy payment, even where a redundancy situation exists.

+ **Minimum Notice and Terms of Employment Acts 1973-2005:** Set out the amount of notice you are entitled to prior to the termination of employment.

+ **Unfair Dismissals Acts 1977-2015:** Circumstances in which unfair dismissal can occur are where your employer terminates your contract of employment, with or without notice, or you terminate your contract of employment, with or without notice, due to the conduct of your employer. This is known as constructive dismissal.

+ **Payment of Wages Act 1991:** Gives employees the right to a payslip showing their gross wages and details of any deductions.

+ **Terms of Employment (Information) Acts 1994-2014:** Within this act it states that employers have a duty to provide each new employee with a written statement of terms within the first two months of starting the job. Information should include: a written contract, information about policies/procedures, rate of pay, hours of work, sick pay and a job description.

+ **Safety and Health at Work Act 2005:** Replaced the Safety and Health at Work Act 1989. Includes employer and employee duties and fines for breaches in relation to safety legislation in the workplace.

+ **Protection of Young Persons (Employment) Act 1996:** Designed to protect the health of young workers and ensure that work carried out during school years does not put young people's education at risk.

+ **Organisation of Working Time Act 1997:** Regulates several employment conditions including maximum working hours, night work, annual leave and public holiday leave.

+ **Freedom of Information Acts 1997-2003:** The right for a member of the public to access records held by public bodies, to have inaccurate personal information material on file corrected, and obtain reasons for decisions affecting oneself.

+ **Freedom of Information Act 2014:** Repeals the 1997 and 2003 Acts. The same statutory rights apply to individuals as the 1997 and 2003 Acts. A number of other changes were introduced which included the widening of the range of bodies to which the FOI legislation applies – it now applies to all public bodies, unless they are specifically exempt.

✚ **Employment Equality Acts 1998–2015:** Prohibits discrimination in a range of employment-related areas. The prohibited grounds of discrimination are gender, civil status, family status, age, race, religion, disability, sexual orientation and membership of the Traveller community.

✚ **Protection of Employees (Part-Term Work) Act 2001:** Prevents discrimination against part-time workers.

✚ **Carer's Leave Act 2001:** Provides for an employee's entitlement to avail of temporary unpaid carer's leave so they can care for someone who requires full-time care and attention.

✚ **Protection of Employees (Fixed-Term Work) Act 2003:** Protects fixed-term employees by ensuring that they cannot be treated less favourably than comparable permanent workers.

✚ **Maternity Protection (Amendment) Act 2004:** Includes provisions relating to ante-natal classes, maternity leave, breastfeeding as well as additional maternity leave, the right to return to work after maternity leave as well as health and safety during, and immediately after, pregnancy.

✚ **Adoptive Leave Act 2005:** Adoptive leave from employment generally for the mother and her right to return to work following such leave.

✚ **Parental Leave (Amendment) Act 2006:** Periods of unpaid leave for parents to care for their children, and for a limited right to paid leave in circumstances of serious family illness known as force majeure.

✚ **Protection of Employment (Temporary Agency Work) Act 2012:** Provides that all temporary agency workers must be treated equally in respect of the duration of working time, rest periods, night work, annual leave, public holidays and pay.

✚ **Protected Disclosures Act 2014:** Protects employees from penalisation if they make a disclosure about wrongdoing in the workplace.

✚ **Equality (Miscellaneous Provisions) Act 2015:** Makes significant amendments to the Employment Equality Act 1998 in the areas of retirement and age discrimination, discrimination by religious, medical and education institutions on religious grounds and indirect discrimination.

✚ **Workplace Relations Act 2015:** Establishes the Workplace Relations Commission (WRC).

✚ **Paternity Leave and Benefit Act 2016:** Allows for statutory paternity leave of two weeks. This must be taken in the first six months following the birth or adoption of a child.

✚ **Mediation Act 2017:** Allows employees to use mediation for certain civil claims e.g. personal injuries actions.

✚ **Data Protection Act 2018 and General Data Protection Regulation (GDPR) 2018:** The General Data Protection Regulation significantly changes data protection law in Europe. It gives you more control over your data. There are higher standards for data protection and the possibilities for penalties if companies are in breach of this.

✚ **Employment (Miscellaneous Provisions) Act 2018:** Bans zero-hour contracts in most situations and provides for minimum payments and banded hours. It also states that employers must provide employees with information on the five core terms of employment within five days of them starting work. It came into effect on 4 March 2019 (Citizens Information).

For further information on all legislation go to www.citizensinformation.ie.

Employee Entitlements

The current employment entitlements relevant to employees in Ireland are as follows:

+ Minimum wage

+ Maximum working week

+ Statement of terms and conditions

+ Statement of pay

+ Breaks during working hours

+ Leave from work

+ Safety in the workplace

+ Equal treatment in the workplace

+ Privacy and data protection

+ Redundancy and dismissal

+ Minimum notice periods

+ Redundancy and dismissal

+ How to make a complaint

+ Where to make a complaint.

Source: www.citizensinformation.ie

chapter 6

THE MULTIDISCIPLINARY TEAM (MDT)

What Is a Team?

A team is a group of people working together towards a common goal. A team works together sharing knowledge, skills and responsibilities in order to achieve whatever their objective is. Some examples of teams are:

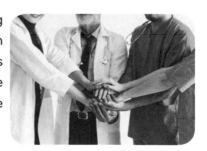

+ Sports teams – GAA, football, basketball, netball

+ Workplace teams

+ Events committees

+ Management teams

+ Healthcare teams.

What Are the Key Attributes of Teams?

What makes one team effective and another not? Effective teams do not happen by accident, they are comprised of a group of people who:

+ Communicate well with each other

+ Focus on goals and results

+ Contribute their fair share to the teamwork

+ Offer each other support

+ Are diverse in their roles, backgrounds and attitudes

+ Trust other team members

+ Have good leadership qualities.

In healthcare a team is called a Multidisciplinary Team (MDT) or sometimes interdisciplinary team. The MDT involves a range of health professionals performing a variety of specialised functions to meet the needs of the patient following a detailed assessment. This will benefit the team, family members and most importantly the client themselves. The MDT ensures that there is consistently high-quality care where clients can be confident that the staff know how to reach the optimum goal in the delivery of care.

Effective communication is vital; team members must listen to each other, give clear messages and share information with all team members in order to avoid mistakes or omissions which could be detrimental to the client's wellbeing. A team working well together is a positive and rewarding experience for team members and clients alike. A good team builds trust with clients and families and creates a sense of security, competence and productiveness where high-quality care can be administered. The security and confidence built by a

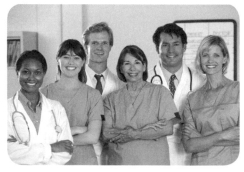

well-functioning team reduces fears and worries that clients and their families may have at critical and often difficult times. A team not working or communicating well brings an insecure and inharmonious atmosphere to a ward, nursing home or other healthcare facility.

Task **Stop and think!**

Think about all the teams you are or have been a member of.

How did the team work together?

Was it a positive or negative experience?

Advantages of Working in a MDT

Multidisciplinary care is essential. It is delivered using a holistic approach, as professionals from a range of disciplines come together to produce a plan of care that will benefit the client and address as many of their needs as possible. The discipline roles may include:

- Doctors
- Nurses
- Physiotherapists
- Speech and language therapists
- Occupational therapists
- Dietitians and nutritionists
- Orthoptists
- Podiatrists
- Psychiatrists.

Each member of the team who specialises in their own area of work will have a different role to play when caring for the client. Advantages of working in an MDT include:

- Improved health outcomes for the client, as a team approach allows for experts and specialists to discuss and plan the best care and treatment options for and with the client
- Enhanced satisfaction for the client as they receive the best care possible

+ Improved morale within the team since no one is working alone or in isolation

+ Goal-orientated work which ensures the client is at the centre of the team's thoughts and efforts

+ Greater collaboration between experts who are able to discuss solutions for individual clients from a range of perspectives.

Members and Roles of a MDT in a Primary Care Setting

Team member	Role
General practitioners (GPs)	GPs play a central role in the delivery of care in the community. They are often the first person that people go to for advice. They provide a broad range of services and can refer a client to specialists in secondary and tertiary centres.
Public health nurses (PHN)	PHNs in Ireland are employed by the HSE to provide a range of healthcare services, for example post-natal care, wound care and palliative care services, in the community for people of all ages. They visit clients in their own home but also see people in clinics in primary healthcare centres.
Physiotherapists	Physiotherapists offer an extensive service to clients with various conditions including difficulties with movement due to illness, injury, ageing or disability. They also help people with heart and lung conditions, neurological conditions and childhood conditions.
Occupational therapists (OT)	OTs focus on helping clients reach and maintain optimum independence through adaptations in the home, Activities of Daily Living (ADLs), environmental adaptations and accessing equipment for the client if necessary.

Team member	Role
Practice nurses	Practice nurses do not do home visits as they are based in GP surgeries and primary care centres. They provide a wide variety of care including immunisations, women's health, ante-natal care, taking blood, health promotion and wound care.
Health Care Assistants	Health Care Assistants assist clients to stay in their own homes for as long as possible by helping with Activities of Daily Living (ADLs) such as washing and dressing, getting in and out of bed and mobilising.
Pharmacists	Pharmacists supply medications to people in the community and are often the first port of call for discussions about minor illnesses to chronic and ongoing health issues.
Chiropodists and podiatrists	Chiropodists and podiatrists are healthcare professionals who have been trained to diagnose and treat abnormal conditions of the feet and lower limbs. They can also treat and alleviate day-to-day foot problems, including toenail problems such as thickened toenails, fungal nail infections and ingrown toenails, corns and calluses.
Community mental health nurses	Community mental health nurses manage a case load and provide services to people with mental health problems including rehabilitation, social skills training, counselling, family support and mental health education.
Speech and language therapists (SALTs)	SALTs provide treatment and care for adults and children who have problems with swallowing and communication.
Dieticians	Dieticians are experts on diet, nutrition and disorders that can be affected by nutrition. They work with clients and doctors to develop individual food plans based on the client's needs.

Members and Roles of a MDT in a Hospital Setting

Team member	Role
Doctors	Doctors in hospitals include consultants, registrars, senior house officers and interns. Consultants have different specialities, for example A&E, vascular, neurology, orthopaedic etc. Their role is to assess clients and refer them to other specialists if necessary.
Nursing team/ clinical nurse specialists	The nursing team in a hospital consists of a director of nursing, an assistant director of nursing, clinical nursing managers plus staff nurses. Within the nursing team are advanced nurse practitioners who may work in A&E, and clinical nurse specialists who may be specialists in areas like diabetes or epilepsy. Healthcare workers would also be part of the nursing team. Their role is to work closely with clients to deliver individualised holistic care.
Physiotherapists	Physiotherapists in hospitals work in their own department but also visit wards and work with clients, for example those who have had a stroke and are unable to mobilise or work, those who require chest physiotherapy.
Speech and language therapists (SALTs)	SALTs in hospitals assess and treat speech, language and communication problems. SALTs also assess clients who have difficulty swallowing and may need a modified diet.
Occupational therapists (OTs)	OTs in hospitals help clients regain, develop or master everyday skills in order to live independent, productive and satisfying lives. They assess clients with physical and mental challenges in order to develop Activities of Daily Living (ADLs) that work best for them.

Team member	Role
Dieticians	Dieticians in hospitals advise clients about nutrition. They develop individual dietary plans, advise on food supplements, weight loss/gain and disorders relating to nutrition.
Medical social workers	Medical social workers in hospitals provide support to clients on a social, practical and emotional level. This could include offering advice about entitlements, counselling and helping a client find housing.
Pharmacists	Pharmacists supply medications to all departments in the hospital and to clients who are being discharged
Chaplain/spiritual advisors	Chaplains and spiritual advisors are available in hospitals for clients with religious and spiritual needs (prayers, last rites, music, poems, chanting, bible readings). Most hospitals will have a chapel or multifaith prayer room.
Discharge co-ordinators	Discharge co-ordinators liaise with the MDT to plan the client's discharge from hospital to home, respite or possibly nursing home care.

(HSE.ie; Power 2019)

TEAMWORK

Team Development: Theories

Working in healthcare involves working as part of a team. You may already have experience of this and have had good and bad experiences. When the team works well it is usually because the right mix of individuals has come together. Unfortunately, when a team doesn't work well, it can become very difficult, cause conflict, low morale and affect the quality of care being delivered. Poor teamwork can be due to poor leadership, personality clashes, lack of time, poor communications, system failures, conflict, lack of balance (everyone wanting to be in charge), lack of rules and low morale (Nifast 2013; Fleming 2004).

In order to work well together, team members need to be able to perform to the best of their ability. Within a team there will be different personalities, each with their own individual traits and characteristics. If they work well together, they can make a very productive and dynamic team that will get the job done to the highest possible standards.

Doctor Meredith Belbin, a UK academic and management consultant who developed the Belbin Team Role Theory in the 1970s, identified that teams with different personality types performed better than teams with fewer personality types. Using his work, managers tasked with organising teams to undertake specific projects have matched team members with recognised roles, resulting in the creation of a successful team which reached the required objective.

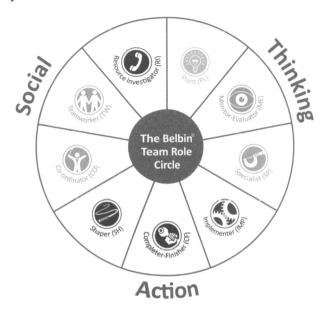

Reproduced with kind permission of Belbin, www.belbin.com

The Nine Team Roles

1. **Co-ordinator:** This person is highly disciplined, controlled and focuses on the objectives. They keep the team focused and are able to get others working to a shared aim. They are confident, mature, good at liaising with others, particularly their fellow team members. (Originally called 'Chairman' by Belbin.)

2. **Shaper:** This individual is dynamic, full of nervous energy, is motivated, energetic, achievement-driven and outgoing. They set challenges and like to be challenged. The shaper helps to shape the team's efforts by trying to put everything together into one single project.

3. **Plant (ideas people):** This person is highly intelligent, an original thinker, generates new ideas and solves difficult problems. They are innovative, inventive, creative and original. They often prefer to work alone.

4. **Monitor-evaluator:** This person can have a dry personality, is intelligent, stable and introverted. They are critical thinkers, and can analyse other people's ideas, weighing up the pros and cons.

5. **Implementer:** This individual has the skills, common sense and ability to organise and put plans into action. They are hardworking and have a systematic approach to work. They are loyal, dependable and practicable.

6. **Resource investigator (developer of ideas):** This individual is creative, can take a new idea from someone else and develop it and would have plenty of contacts outside a team. They are quick, good communicators and networkers who seek and find options. They often need to work with others.

7. **Teamworker:** This person is supportive, sociable and flexible. They make good listeners and are loyal to the team. They build on new ideas as opposed to picking holes in them.

8. **Completer-finisher:** This individual pays attention to detail, is accurate and has high standards. They can, however, be anxious and introvert and find it hard to delegate, but will never miss a deadline.

9. **Specialist:** This individual is a technical expert in their own field. They are highly focused, capable and extremely knowledgeable within their area of expertise. They tend to show little interest in others' work and can be loners (Jay 2003).

Having a team with all the above individuals would be near perfect and probably highly unlikely to achieve. Nonetheless, most people will have two or three characteristics of the above nine roles.

Effective and skilled leaders will identify their team members' roles to establish the right mix and form a well-structured team that will perform well together.

Stop and think!

Can you recognise yourself in any of the above roles?

For further reading on the roles, refer to https://www.belbin.com/about/belbin-team-roles/

Framework for Team Development

A framework for team development was established in the mid 1960s by a psychologist called Bruce Tuckman. The five stages of team development are:

1. **Forming:** Refers to the organisation or the reorganisation of a team which first gets to know each other. They may be anxious about meeting, and no rules or methods of working are established.

2. **Storming:** Members start to grow in confidence as they start to feel comfortable in their roles. There can be disagreements and a certain amount of infighting is normal.

3. **Norming:** Now the group moves on to establish norms, standards and ground rules. Roles have been established and people offer support to each other. This process is needed as the pressure builds to produce results.

4. **Performing:** This is when the team is getting the job done, the group is more united and performing as a team in an enthusiastic way. People feel secure enough to speak out and give their opinions.

5. **Adjourning:** This is when the task is complete and the group separates.

Being a Team Member

Stop and think!

Write down all the teams you have been involved in.

What role did you have in the team?

What were the positive and negative aspects of being part of a team?

Being a team member can be rewarding. When the team gels or works well together, members can derive a great sense of satisfaction. Working together towards a common goal means everyone is pulling together for the same thing, and in healthcare the goal is to provide the best quality care to the clients.

✚ Being a team member means not having to do all the work yourself – the weight of the job doesn't fall to one person.

✚ Being a team member means having someone to talk to when needed; debriefing, having support if your shift hasn't gone well, and sharing problems are all situations where team members can help one another.

✚ Being a team member means having fun, bouncing ideas off one another and brainstorming.

✚ Being a team member can be socially rewarding; some teams get on so well that they may socialise together and, if no one is intentionally left out, this can be a really good way to bond further. Team-building days can also be fun and a way of getting to know people outside of work.

As a team member, it is important to remember to:

✚ Respect each other's opinion even if you don't necessarily agree with it.

✚ Respect diversity and accept each other's culture, religion and individuality.

✚ Be courteous to each other even if you don't get on.

✚ Communicate well and listen to other people.

✚ Try to sort out any conflict that arises between yourselves. If unable to do so, report to a supervisor who should be able to help

✚ Be flexible and help your team members should the need arise e.g. cover shifts for them if you can.

✚ Be honest with your team members if things aren't working or need reviewing.

- Be enthusiastic and approachable.

- Keep any conflict away from clients – they will pick up on it and it can cause discomfort for everyone.

- Welcome new members to the team; remember what it was like to be a new member yourself.

(Fleming 2004; Nifast 2013)

Accepting Guidance and Direction as a Team Member

We all need guidance and direction at times, especially when starting a new job or work experience. We need to be helped in relation to the following:

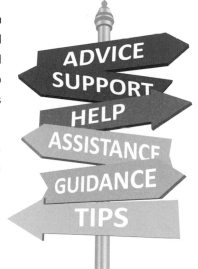

- How the workplace runs – this can include things like being advised about the shift patterns, tea and lunch breaks, what uniform to wear, the training required, who is in charge and who to report to.

- Guidance on rules, regulations, policies and procedures – this can relate to HIQA standards.

- The clients we will be looking after.

- The job we are expected to do – what our role is.

We need to be directed and advised or we might not know where we precisely fit in or if we are doing things correctly. Usually in a new job or work experience, you are assigned a mentor or a buddy who helps direct you, show you where things are and outline the routine.

Guidance, direction and delegation of jobs will also be given by a supervisor or nurse in charge. The nurse will usually delegate the HCA jobs associated with their role e.g. washing and dressing, assisting with eating and drinking etc.

It is important to be aware of tasks that are beyond the role e.g. administrating medication, diagnosing illness, inserting or removing tubes from a person's body, performing procedures that require sterile techniques e.g. dressings or catheterisation. The care assistant should not carry them out, even if asked to, as it risks causing harm to the client (Carter and Goldschmidt 2010).

Accepting guidance and direction is necessary:

+ When starting a new job – guidance and direction from a mentor or supervisor

+ When undertaking a new task e.g. taking observations

+ When developing a new skill e.g. computer skills

+ When mentoring another person.

Receiving Guidance and Direction as a Team Member

+ Listen to the person giving guidance and direction.

+ Be sure to understand what is being said. If you don't, say so.

+ Don't take any constructive criticism personally. It is an observation made by another team member.

+ Ask for specifics if you are unsure about what the person giving guidance is saying.

+ Don't be defensive.

+ Acknowledge the speaker's point of view.

+ Discuss ways of how to improve with the supervisor/person in charge or maybe do reflective practice (see chapter 13).

+ Never perform a task that you have not been taught to do or you are uncomfortable with carrying out.

+ Never ignore a job allocated to you because you don't know how to do it; make sure you ask.

(Everyday Health 2017; Carter and Goldschmidt 2010)

Stop and think!
Who gives guidance and direction in the
healthcare setting?

Who Gives Guidance and Direction?

+ Nurses
+ Doctors
+ Managers
+ Residents
+ Other care assistants
+ Family members
+ Other members of staff in the care
  facility in which are working

Stop and think!
How does it feel to accept guidance and direction?

Is it easy to accept guidance and direction?

What can you gain from accepting guidance and direction?

When can it become difficult?

Case Study: **Andrew and Aoife**

Andrew has just started a job as a HCA on Ward 6 – a busy
medical ward. He is very nervous. He has arrived on the
ward and is greeted by the senior nurse and Aoife, who is a
senior HCA and has been allocated to be his mentor for the
day. Aoife shows Andrew where to put his coat and bag and
explains how the ward runs. Aoife then shows Andrew
around the ward including the store cupboard, the kitchen
and the sluice room. She informs him about break times and
advises him to stick with her 'like glue' today until he finds
his feet. They go to the nurses station for handover where
Aoife introduces Andrew to the rest of the team.

What are the good examples of guidance and direction here?

How do you think Andrew feels by the time he starts listening to handover?

Receiving Feedback

Receiving feedback is very important and valuable. It is essential for personal and professional growth. When we receive feedback, it means we are being given information about our performance. We can receive feedback for different aspects of our life e.g. work or college. It can help us to recognise the areas that we are doing well in and those we need to work on. Feedback can help to identify the ways in which we can develop the areas that require improvement e.g. by going on courses to update our skills.

Receiving feedback is a part of quality assurance and improvement and is essential when it comes to delivering excellent care in the clinical environment. Giving and receiving feedback at times may not be easy. People can take things to heart and find the feedback difficult. Positive feedback can improve our performance. It can build morale, help to identify potential problems before they arise, build confidence, help to identify training needs and promote best practice (Nifast 2013).

There are different types of feedback:

Informal: This is done on a day-to-day basis and is usually given verbally. It can be done by colleagues.

Formal: This is usually carried out in a formal setting with a manager. It is written feedback.

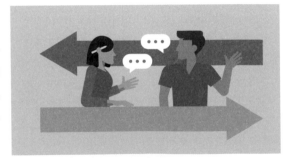

The employee should find out what the policy is in the place of work in relation to formal feedback sessions, which are often called appraisals.

Formative: This is carried out when a student is undertaking a course. It is usually done at a time during the course when the student has acquired a new skill or written an assignment. The learner is offered the opportunity to receive feedback so they can be given advice where to improve things if necessary.

Summative: This is usually the end part of a course when a student completes a skills demonstration or an assignment and they are given a mark, together with written feedback. (Hardavella et al. 2017)

Healthcare staff should recognise that receiving feedback ought not to be a negative experience. Instead it should be used as a tool for learning. Feedback should be 'constructive, accurate, factual, impersonal, focused on targets, morale boasting, and options for improvement should be given' (Nifast 2013).

Feedback can be given by different people

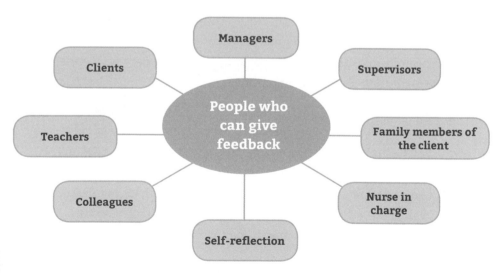

In the healthcare setting, if feedback is not given and accepted it could be detrimental to client care. Staff may carry on working, thinking that they are performing perfectly well, when perhaps they are not as competent as they believe they are or, for some reason, their standards have slipped (Hardavella et al. 2017).

When receiving feedback, it is helpful to remember the following:

+ Adopt an open-minded approach.

+ Listen carefully to what is being said.

+ Don't become defensive.

+ Be willing to change.

+ Ask questions when the person has finished speaking.

+ Ask how you can improve your performance.

+ If you think of something after the feedback session that you would like to discuss with your supervisor, make a follow-up appointment.

+ View it as a way of reflecting on your strengths and on how to improve your confidence in the area you are working in.

+ Think positively and be proactive e.g. be ready to apply for an appropriate course.

+ Embrace the feedback session and use it as a learning experience.

(Hardavella et al. 2017)

Case Study: Patrick and Jo

Patrick and Jo are working together in a nursing home. Patrick has only been working there for three weeks. They go for break together and Jo says to Patrick, 'Patrick, you have been working really hard lately. The nurse in charge will be really pleased with you; you were so kind to Mrs Mallon this morning when you got her that extra cup of tea.'

What kind of feedback was displayed in this case study?

Case Study: Students' and first assessment brief

Fifteen students are undertaking the Care Support Module as part of the QQI Level 5 Healthcare Support Certificate. Their tutor has given them their first assessment brief which is a learner record. They have been given a date by which they should hand draft work in to be given feedback by the tutor.

What kind of feedback do you think the students may receive?

chapter 8

BUILDING CLIENT RELATIONSHIPS

Professional Relationships with Clients

Working within the healthcare profession is about being part of a widely recognised and trusted team of people. As a HCA, it is important to remember that the client and the family expect a level of care where the team are acting in their best interest and treating them with dignity and respect. Professional standards must be maintained, and it is important for HCAs to be aware of professional boundaries so as not to jeopardize the therapeutic nurse–patient relationship. One way to maintain a professional relationship with clients is to have boundaries.

Boundaries

What is a boundary? Something that indicates a limit. A marker? A line not to be crossed?

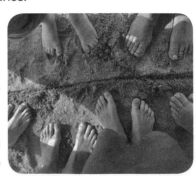

Sometimes a boundary is visible e.g. a boundary between two countries where there is a border, or a wall indicating a farmer's land. On the other hand, a boundary can be invisible, for example between a teacher and a student, or a manager and a worker.

The relationship between a healthcare worker and client is therapeutic in nature; it is built on trust, respect, professional intimacy, empathy and power (College of Nurses of Ontario 2006). The relationship is also unequal as the carer is privy to personal and confidential information about the client which can leave the client in a vulnerable position.

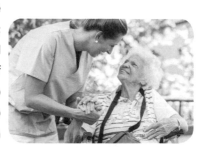

Professional Boundaries in Nursing		
Under-Involved	**Zone of Helpfulness**	**Over-Involved**
Distance yourself in an effort not to 'get too close'		Discuss your personal or intimate information
Fail to meet the client's needs		Tell or keep clients' secrets
		Assume role of 'super nurse'
Spend more time with staff than clients		Spend time with clients outside of work hours

(*Adapted from:* National Council of State Boards of Nursing (NCSBN). (2018). *A Nurse's Guide to Professional Boundaries.* Chicago, IL: NCSBN.)

Healthcare workers must be aware that the relationships with clients and their families are professional relationships where boundaries apply. They must make sure not to cross these boundaries and break the therapeutic relationship with the client. On some occasions, unintentionally and through no harm, boundaries may be blurred or crossed e.g. accepting a very generous expensive gift from a client or becoming over-involved in their care. The other extreme is if the boundaries are violated e.g. having a sexual relationship with a client or stealing from them. Carers and nurses can become either under- or over-involved with their clients which is where the issues regarding professional boundaries can become blurred. The goal is to stay within the middle section – the zone of helpfulness.

Examples of the differences between professional and personal relationships include the following:

Professional	Personal
Time-bound, limited by the client's need for nursing care; carer's hours of work are also taken in consideration	Personal choice for length of relationship – it may last a lifetime
Carer has a distinct role and purpose when caring for the client	No specific role definition in a friendship
Structured and guided by regulations, codes of practice and professional standards	No structure – guided by personal and common interests, values and beliefs
Trained, formal knowledge and preparation for care delivery	No training or formal knowledge necessary
Responsible for welfare of the person	Equal responsibility
Carer paid to provide care	No payment made in a friendship
Relationship defined and limited to healthcare settings e.g. hospital, nursing home, home care	Relationship can take place anywhere e.g. own home
Power balance is unequal: the carer is privy to confidential information about the client	Relationship is relatively equal
Purpose of the relationship is to provide care, goal-directed, meet the needs of a client	Relationship is unstructured, spontaneous and pleasurable

(*Adapted from:* BCRS now VHHSC. 1992 and NCSBN 2018. *A Nurse's Guide to Professional Boundaries;* Milgram 1992; RNBC 2006.)

Task

Stop and think!

After what you have read and learnt about boundaries, using the diagram on page 65, where in the zone of helpfulness do the following actions fit?

+ Visiting a client on your day off
+ Treating all clients all the time with dignity and respect
+ Being professional in the way you speak, act and dress at work
+ Being respectful to clients and their family members
+ Maintaining confidentiality
+ Discussing your intimate or personal issues with a client or their family members
+ Including the client as a partner in his/her care
+ Ensuring good communication pathways with the client and family members
+ Keeping secrets for a client or with a client
+ Engaging in a relationship of a sexual nature with a client
+ Ignoring a client's cry for help
+ Accepting money from a client or a family member
+ Frequently thinking about a client when away from work
+ Giving a client personal contact details unless required as part of your job
+ Showing no interest in the client of family member
+ Providing only the very basic level of care
+ Showing very little or no empathy
+ Not listening to the client
+ Being an advocate for the client (speaking up for them when they need it)
+ Respecting the client's decisions and choices

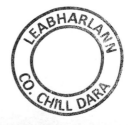

A Final Thought to Consider about Boundaries

Although we must have professional boundaries when we are nursing people, there are times when these may be unintentionally crossed, and we must question whether this is wrong. In some healthcare settings, hospices, home care environments and nursing homes, to name a few, clients can become more like family members as we nurse them over a long period of time. We may nurse them until they die or until we change jobs, and we feel sad when they die or when we say goodbye. Is it so wrong for us to feel this way?

As carers we are human beings, we have feelings and although we are in a position of trust and, some may say, power, we do develop meaningful relationships with some clients and their families where the boundaries may not necessarily be crossed but slightly blurred. How can we be expected to walk out the door and stop thinking about someone for whom we care who is dying? How can we be expected to remain unaffected or uninspired by a client of ours battling with a long-term illness and their unrelenting positivity in the face of adversity. What we must do is be aware that we can't take everyone with us on our journey. Some clients we will remember, and sometimes the boundaries may be crossed slightly, but they should never be crossed to the point where the person has been violated and where we have abused our position of trust.

Interpersonal Skills in Care Work

Task **Stop and think!**
What are interpersonal skills?

As a HCA, why do I need to enhance my interpersonal skills?

How am I interpersonally skilled?

'Interpersonal' relates to the interaction between people. Having inter-personal skills is having the ability to deal with others. In care work, having interpersonal skills is so important. As a HCA you will be taking care of clients who are vulnerable due to illness, disability or age factors. You will

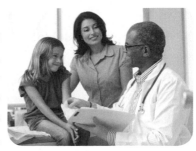

also be communicating and interacting with those clients' family members. Finally, you will be a part of a multi-disciplinary team (MDT) and you will be expected to work together with this group of people in the best interest of the clients. Having good interpersonal skills will develop these relationships. Clients and their family will develop trust in you, and the MDT will see you as a valued member of the team who can be relied upon and trusted.

> **Task** **Stop and think!**
> List the types of interpersonal skills used on a day-to-day basis.

Interpersonal skills can be:

- ✦ **Having a good attitude:** Being friendly, kind, warm and open

- ✦ **Engaging in teamwork:** Working as part of a team, pulling your weight

- ✦ **Showing empathy:** Putting yourself in another's shoes, seeing things from their perspective and trying to understand what they are going through

- ✦ **Having a sense of humour:** Seeing the lighter side of things, not taking things too seriously, being appropriate with humour

- ✦ **Showing compassion:** Having feelings for clients, colleagues, family members, being there for them when they need you

- ✦ **Being tactful:** Keeping things private, not gossiping

- ✦ **Being respectful:** Valuing your clients, family members and colleagues

- ✦ **Having cultural awareness:** Being open to and learning about different cultures

- ✦ **Being non-judgemental:** Not judging anyone no matter what their opinions, beliefs or morals are

+ **Being dependable:** Being able to be relied upon by colleagues and clients

+ **Having patience:** Being calm and gentle in your approach

+ **Listening actively:** Listening to others to gain information; for example, when a client is upset and you want to find out why they are upset, you may need to listen to hear more than the words they are speaking.

+ **Being courteous:** Being polite and kind to colleagues, clients and family

+ **Being aware of verbal and non-verbal communication:** Talking to people and using appropriate body language

(Duffy 2008; McCorry and Mason 2011)

Interpersonal skills in care work are essential. They can be learnt and developed over time. You may already have some of the interpersonal skills listed above. Having a sense of self and knowing who you are is important when it comes to interpersonal skills, and using reflective practice can help to develop our interpersonal skills (see Chapter 13). We can reflect on situations that occur in work or in work experience and see how our interpersonal skills are developing over time.

Ultimately, part of the role of a HCA is to have excellent interpersonal skills in order to deliver exceptional quality care to clients and to work as part of a team.

At times interpersonal issues may arise in the workplace. These issues can involve the client, family members or colleagues. Interpersonal issues can be challenging but can also be a learning experience.

Task

Stop and think!
List as interpersonal issues that can arise in care work.

Discuss what problems these issues could cause.

What can you learn from them?

Interpersonal issues that can arise in care work include:

+ **Conflict with the client:** Clients who are feeling vulnerable and don't wish to be looked after, clients who make a complaint, conflict over long waiting times

+ **Conflict with family members:** Families feeling worried and anxious about their loved one and taking their fears out on you, people who make a complaint

+ **Conflict with a colleague/colleagues:** Clashes in personality, differences of opinion

+ **Cultural and religious diversity:** Differences in beliefs/opinions, lack of understanding about a person's needs

+ **Language barriers:** Difficulties in communicating with clients causing frustration and annoyance

+ **Behavioural challenges:** Clients whose behaviour challenges us e.g. aggression, confusion, dementia. Lack of training in this area can cause problems for the client and the care worker. Not knowing how to communicate and care for a client whose behaviour is challenging can be frightening and worrying, leaving the care worker feeling vulnerable and unable to communicate effectively with the client.

+ **Communication challenges:** Clients who are unable to communicate verbally due to a condition such as stroke may have difficulty voicing their needs to the healthcare team, which can lead to frustration.

+ **Becoming part of a team:** Changes in the team, getting to know team members, learning to work as part of a team, communication skills, possible conflict within a team

Relationships with Family, Visitors and Significant Others

Task Stop and think!
What is the meaning of family to you?

Are you a member of a family?

Who is in your family?

Family can be whoever the client says it is; it doesn't always have to be a blood relative. The client's significant other may be a best friend or a neighbour. We will come across clients who have very large families and always seem to have someone visiting and we will come across some who have no one. Sometimes families can be estranged: never judge, as each family is different and we don't know what the situation is. A client might tell you that they have a daughter who never visits them; it is not our place to judge the daughter as we don't know why she never visits. Families come in all different shapes and sizes.

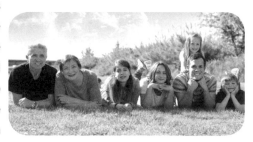

Task Stop and think!
Can you name different types of families?

Family Types

+ **Nuclear family:** A married or co-habitational couple with children

+ **Nuclear dyad family:** A couple with no children

+ **Extended family:** A nuclear family with close relatives such as grandparents, aunts and uncles

+ **Step/blended family:** Divorced, separated or widowed parents with children who form new families with a new partner

+ **Adoptive family:** A family where one or more of the children has been adopted

+ **Same-sex family:** A family where one or more of the members are lesbian, gay, bisexual or transgender (LGBT), and/or where children are raised by an opposite-sex couple where at least one partner is LGBT

+ **Single-parent family:** A lone parent raising one or more children on their own

(Giddens 2001)

Visitors and Significant Others

When meeting visitors in any care setting it is important to be courteous, respectful and kind. A smile goes a long way. At times we may meet people who might not be respectful towards us, but we must remember that they may be going through difficult situations that might be affecting their behaviour e.g. bereavement, difficult news or family arguments. It is important not to take anything that is said personally; but having said that, you are not expected to tolerate any form of abuse.

Task Stop and think!
How do you think a visitor may feel about their loved one being admitted to a care facility?

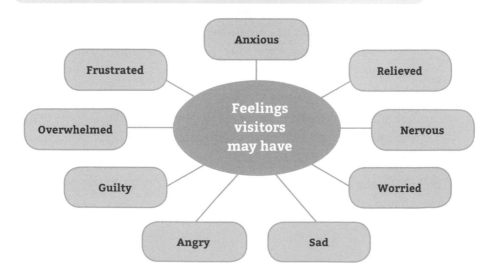

Caring for Visitors and Significant Others

Task   **Stop and think!**
How can the HCA and MDT care for
the client's significant others?

The client's loved ones want the best for them. Staff want to provide the best care. Therefore it is important for everyone working together to keep in mind that the client is at the centre of this approach.

By getting to know the client's significant others and having an open channel of communication, a good relationship can be built. The following are ways to help and support significant others:

+ If the client gives consent, the nurse can include the next of kin in the care planning process.

+ Ask them about the client – after all, they know them the best.

+ If the client wishes, include the significant others in their care e.g. assisting with mealtimes.

+ If the client can go out, encourage the significant others to take them out.

+ Have open, honest communication with the significant others.

+ Ensure the significant others are aware of visiting times. Nursing homes generally have open visiting times. Find out what the policy is. Some times of the day are busier than others e.g. morning times and mealtimes. Hospitals may have more rigid visiting times depending on the ward.

+ Allow for privacy during visiting. Sometimes communal areas do not allow for privacy, in which case you can facilitate by assisting the client back to their room or encouraging the significant others to take them out (Nazarko 2000).

+ Refer any concerns significant others may have to the person in charge.

(Adapted from Nova Scotia College of Nursing, 2019; CARNA, 2011 and Milgram, 1992 cited in British Columbia College of Nursing Professionals, 2019)

Case Study: Emma and Edith

Edith is a 75-year-old lady who is being admitted to the nursing home in which you work. Edith has numerous health problems but the main reason she is being admitted is because she has dementia. Edith was being cared for by her daughter Emma in Emma's house, however Edith is deteriorating quite quickly, and it was decided by the family that Edith now needs 24-hour care. You are helping the nurse get Edith settled and Emma is with her. You notice Emma asking the nurse lots of questions such as 'When can I visit?', 'What kind of food is available?', 'Will I be able to help my mother get dressed in the morning?', 'Can my mother have her favourite blanket?' Emma seems agitated and restless.

What do you think might be happening for Emma at this time?

How can you and the nurse help Emma?

Emma might be feeling very anxious about the decision to admit her mother into long-term care. She may also be feeling guilty that she is not able to look after her mother in her home anymore. Emma is asking questions looking for reassurance about the care her mother will receive, therefore the most important thing is to reassure Emma.

After settling Edith, the nurse may spend time with Emma explaining how the nursing home runs, letting her know that she can get involved in her mother's care if her mother wishes. Emma will be reassured that the staff are there to give the best quality of care to Edith. Good, open, honest communication with family members is very important to make them feel part of the care provided and prevent upset and possible complaints.

Verbal and Non-Verbal Communication in the Care Environment

Effective communication is one of the most important and vital skills a healthcare worker can possess. As a HCA you will be working alongside clients, family members and staff members and you will always be expected to communicate successfully with them. If just one link in the communication chain is broken, the quality of care given to the patient can suffer. Communication is a dynamic and complex process that helps to establish relationships, 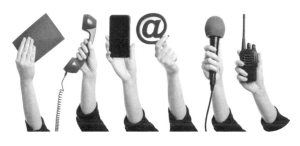 share information and ideas, and give meaning to everything we do. Miscommunication, on the other hand, can lead to complaints and misunderstandings. For example, incorrect information passed from one member of the team to another or information not passed on at all could jeopardize the care of the client.

Effective communication in healthcare settings is important as a major contribution to:

+ Assessing the client

+ Formulating a plan of care and treatment

+ Passing information between MDTs

+ Developing relationships

+ Passing information to clients and family members

+ Helping clients and family members understand existing and changing plans of care/treatment

+ Ensuring client satisfaction with the care being provided

+ Reassuring clients

+ Promoting trust within healthcare/client relationships

+ Ensuring better client outcome.

The Process of Communication

Communication is a two-way process. Communicating is not just telling someone something (giving information), it is also about listening and observing (receiving information).

Communication involves at least two people: a sender and a receiver.

✚ The sender is the person who has the information to share e.g. the HCA telling the client that they can have a wash if they want one.

✚ The receiver is the person for whom the information is intended e.g. the client.

✚ The sender delivers the information in the form of a message which the receiver may or may not understand, in this case, verbal communication (the spoken word).

✚ Through feedback, or a return message, the receiver lets the sender know whether the message was received and understood. In this case the client can non-verbally respond by nodding or shaking their head, or can verbally respond by saying yes or no.

✚ The sender knows the message has been delivered.

The process of communication can be affected by many different things. This is known as noise, which can literally be 'noise' as in sound, but can be other things as well:

✚ **Environmental noise:** Such as phones ringing, people talking, loud televisions or radios.

✚ **Physical noise:** The person may be hungry or tired and stop listening to the information they are being given.

✚ **Psychological noise:** The person may be feeling upset about something or even depressed which can interfere with the listening process.

✚ **Cultural noise:** Coming from different backgrounds with different values, knowledge and belief systems may mean that unfamiliar sounds can be distracting or uncomfortable to be near.

+ **Language barriers:** Different accents and dialects may be hard to understand.

+ **Lack of privacy:** Clients may not wish to tell a healthcare professional personal information if there is only a curtain between them and the client next to them.

+ **Constant interruptions:** If during an assessment, the doctor or nurse talking to the client is constantly interrupted, the client may start to feel that their information can't be of much value or importance.

+ **Impaired vision:** Clients may not be able to read information given to them about conditions or medication.

+ **Impaired hearing:** A client may not hear important information that is being given to them e.g. the date of their next appointment or even information about medication.

+ **Non-verbal communication:** This can be misinterpreted depending on culture e.g. eye contact.

+ **Medical jargon:** This refers to the way healthcare professionals communicate with each other; a client may not understand the terminology being used.

+ **Staffing shortages:** Staff shortages can lead to staff rushing to 'get the job done', and clients may therefore feel that they can't talk to the staff and don't want to bother them as they are too busy.

+ **Lack of training:** All HCAs working with clients suffering with dementia will require specific training on how to communicate effectively with dementia clients taking all environmental factors into consideration.

+ **Fear of upsetting the client:** Sometimes healthcare workers may be afraid of saying the wrong thing and upsetting the client, or even being asked a difficult question.

Physical Disabilities and Communication

CVA Cerebrovascular Accident (Stroke)	Aphasia (sometimes referred to as dysphasia) – the most common language disorder caused by stroke. It affects understanding, speech, reading and writing Receptive aphasia – difficulty in understanding what is being said Expressive aphasia – understands all that is being said, but may not be able to speak (communicates through sounds) Dysarthria – weakness of the speaking muscles which means the client may have difficulty speaking clearly (Stroke Association Information Service 2012)
Dementia	Creates difficulties in the part of the brain that controls memory and speech
Parkinson's Disease	Creates difficulties with speech and communication from memory problems, difficulties in making facial expressions, speaking slowly and quietly (Parkinsons UK)
Multiple Sclerosis	Can cause dysarthria which is a problem with physically producing the sounds of speech but with no problems in understanding, reading or writing (unless another physical problem, such as arthritic fingers, affects these)
Motor Neurone Disease	Can cause dysarthria. Speech and language therapy may improve the speech of some clients with dysarthria. The success of treatment will depend on the extent and location of the brain damage or dysfunction, the underlying condition causing it, and the individual's personal circumstances.

| Deafness | Complete or partial. Some people are born deaf and some develop deafness as they grow older. Other reasons include genetic disorders or damage to the ear drum. It can be temporary if, for example, it is caused by an ear infection or a build-up of wax. |
| Visual impairment | Different types of visual impairments from partial sightedness to full blindness. Common causes of sight loss include age-related macular degeneration, cataract, glaucoma and diabetic retinopathy. |

Case Study: Mrs Murphy

Mrs Murphy has been admitted to the busy medical ward you work on following a suspected stroke. She is having difficulty with her speech and is becoming increasingly frustrated and angry because staff are having difficulty understanding what she is trying to say. Mrs Murphy rings her call bell and you go into her to see what she would like. She tries to tell you something, but you are struggling to understand. In the end she smacks her hand off the bed and turns her head away from you.

How do you think Mrs Murphy is feeling in this situation?

What can you do to help her?

What aids to communication could help Mrs Murphy?

Ways to Communicate Effectively

+ Sit down next to the person and introduce yourself.
+ Explain the purpose of your being there.
+ Use simple, clear language.
+ Use short sentences giving only one piece of information at a time.
+ Only ask one question at a time.

+ Encourage the individual to speak and ask questions to which you know the answer so you can assess the client's speech pattern.

+ Use gestures.

+ Encourage the individual to use gestures.

+ Encourage an individual who requires glasses to wear them.

+ If a client has a visual impairment, give them very clear, direct instructions when helping them e.g. 'the chair is right behind you'.

+ Ensure the individual who requires a hearing aid is wearing it unless they don't wish to do so.

+ If a client is deaf, avoid approaching them from behind, as this may startle them.

+ If they can hear on one side, speak to them on that side.

+ Do not cover your mouth when speaking to them as they may be able to lip read. In any case, covering your mouth will cause your words to be muffled and unclear.

+ Listen, be patient and wait for a response.

+ Use aids to communication if they have them.

Aids to Communication

There are many aids to assist HCA–client communication, namely Augmentative and Alternative Communication (AAC) Products such as scanning communication aids, sequential communication aids, auditory (hearing) communication aids and tactile (touch) communication aids (Amy Speech and Language Therapy 2010).

Task **Activity**
This can be done in the classroom setting or outside.

1. Pair up, with Person A to be blindfolded and Person B to be the guide.

2. Person B (the guide) must give very clear instructions and guide Person A (the blindfolded person) either around the room or on a short walk outside.

3. Person A can hold onto Person B if they feel unsteady.

4. Now swap roles and repeat the activity.

5. Following the activity, discuss the following:

   (a) How did you feel being 'blind'?

   (b) How did you feel leading your partner around the room/ outside?

   (c) Think about how a client with a visual impairment may feel who has been admitted into a care facility for the first time.

Non-Verbal Communication

Much of what we communicate is done through non-verbal communication or body language. We may have already communicated something to our client before we have spoken to them. A look can often reveal more accurately what we are thinking than words can. As HCAs it is important to be aware of your non-verbal communication and to be aware of your clients.

Task **Stop and think!**
What are the signs of non-verbal communication?

Look around at all the people you can see now and see what non-verbal signs they are displaying.

+ **Posture/position:** This is how we stand or sit. Are we standing tall or slouching? Are we facing the person or walking away from them? Face-to-face communication is the most common interaction we have with clients and members of the multidisciplinary team and this lends itself to positive interactions. If we are facing away from them when communicating, it can be thought of as being rude and suggest that we are not really interested. Our words may also not carry clearly enough to be heard or understood.

+ **Facial expressions:** Facial expressions say a lot: a smile or a frown can express joy, sadness, pain. We can read the client's facial expressions when observing and assessing them. For example, they might grimace when they are being moved which could indicate they are in pain. This would need to be reported to the person/nurse in charge immediately. It is important to be aware of our own facial expressions as clients will be able to read them; for example, if we are assisting them with changing a colostomy bag or changing a continence pad where there may be an unpleasant smell, it is important to be mindful that they may see us reacting to the smell, and this can cause embarrassment for the client.

+ **Gestures:** Include movement of the head, hands, eyes and other body parts. They often are used instead of words but can accompany words too. Examples can be gestures indicating that we would like someone to stop, wait, come here, be quiet or shush.

+ **Eye contact:** Can indicate that a person is listening, while a lack of eye contact or looking away from someone when they are talking can be seen as avoidance or being disinterested.

+ **Appropriate touch:** Can include gently holding someone's hand with their consent if they are upset, which can give great comfort and is appropriate in the healthcare setting.

+ **Distance/personal space:** Everyone has a personal space, and if that space is invaded, a person can feel threatened and anxious. As HCAs you will need to go into people's personal space to carry out care, but you must always gain consent before doing so. An example might be, 'Is it okay if I help you with a wash this morning?' Always treat the person with respect and recognise their need for privacy.

Active Listening

Active listening is part of communicating with people. To show you are listening to someone you must give them your full attention. If possible, sit down with the person and maintain eye contact. Give them time to speak and don't interrupt them. Nod and give non-verbal feedback where appropriate. When they have said what they want to say, you can paraphrase – meaning that you can repeat what the person has said back to them but in your own words. This is an excellent communication skill to have as it shows you have understood the message that has been given. It is a useful tool to confirm back an instruction relating to a client between team members.

Listening to someone makes them feel as though you really care about what they are saying, that you will help them and take care of them. It helps to build a trusting relationship and make a client feel safe in your care.

Task   **Activity**

With a partner, where Person A is the HCA and Person B is a client, act out the following scenario: Person B has been admitted to a medical ward following a diagnosis of diabetes, and they have many worries and want to talk. Person B is explaining those worries to Person A.

Person A needs to use their listening skills without interrupting Person B and paraphrase Person B's worries back to them.

Swap roles and have Person A do the talking with Person B listening.

+ How did it feel to be listened to?

+ How did it feel to listen without interrupting?

+ How can you use this scenario in work or on work experience?

Remember

+ Verbal and non-verbal communication in healthcare settings is a vital part of client care.

+ As a HCA you will communicate with clients, family members and members of the MDT.

+ Miscommunication can lead to complaints and jeopardize client safety.

+ Communication is a two-way process.

+ There are many things that can get in the way of the communication process e.g. noise, lack of information and lack of training.

+ Aids to communication are available to help people who have communication difficulties. Ask the person/nurse in charge what is available in your place of work.

+ Remember to be aware of your non-verbal communication: not only are you observing your clients and their family members, but they are observing you too.

Active listening is a vital part of your job. Practise how to do it and remember how respectful it feels to be listened to.

chapter 9

PLANNING AND DELIVERING QUALITY CARE

Confidentiality and Client Information

All residents and clients in healthcare have a fundamental right to expect their personal details to be kept private and confidential. Confidentiality is central to client care. The client should be confident that personal information will not be passed on, unless there is a professional reason for doing so (Nolan 2003).

The confidentiality bond between healthcare professionals and clients is not new. It has been enshrined in legal and professional codes of practice for many years and has been included in contracts of employment (O'Dowd 2009; IHF 2013).

Relevant information about clients' health problems will, at times, obviously need to be passed between the MDT members e.g. between doctors, nurses, HCAs, physiotherapists, occupational therapists and dieticians to name but a few. However, the information shared should be relevant only to the appropriate and relevant MDT member e.g. the physiotherapist looking after a client following a stroke may be focusing only on that client's physical needs. They will not need to know about the difficulties members of the client's family are having, unless there is a direct link to or bearing on the health problems of the client.

Sometimes, however, a client will give you information and ask you not to tell anyone about it e.g that they are being abused psychologically, physically or even sexually. This would then become **a safeguarding issue**. In these circumstances you are obliged and duty-bound to inform a senior staff member so they can carry out the correct procedures to help that person. There are some situations where legally, nurses and other health practitioners can breach client confidentiality. These are:

+ Where the client may be harmed

+ Notifying relevant authorities of an infectious disease

+ When ordered to by a judge

+ Where another person may be harmed

+ In instances of child protection issues.

(inmo.ie – Paul McGinn Legal Dialogue: Confidentiality issues)

The role of the HCA is to reassure the client that such confidential information will only be given to a person who can be absolutely trusted to maintain confidentilaity, and then inform the nurse in charge of any of the situations above and leave it to the nurse to deal with.

Confidentiality Case Studies

Case Study 1: You work in a local nursing home in a small village. One day you go to the shop and a lady you know stops you and asks, 'How's Mrs Jones doing? I hear she's with you in the nursing home'. You are caught off guard but what do you do?

Case Study 2: You are a care worker in a busy medical ward. You notice a nurse attending on a doctor's ward round leave a client's medical folder open on a bed where other clients can see it. The nurse then leaves the six-bedded room without the folder and carries on with the ward round. What do you do?

Case Study 3: Two staff members are in the hospital canteen discussing Mr Armstrong who is critically ill on their ward. They are telling a friend of theirs who works on another ward about Mr Armstrong's personal issues and why he has ended up in hospital. What they don't realise is that a member of Mr Armstrong's family is sitting at the table next to them and has overheard everything. What could happen in this situation? Are the staff members wrong? What should you do?

Possible Solutions

Case Study 1: It would be easy to say to the lady in the shop that yes, Mrs Jones *is* in the nursing home and is settling in nicely, however, maybe Mrs Jones doesn't want anyone to know she is in the nursing home, so we must be very careful here. The best thing to do would be to say something like, 'I'm really sorry but I can't discuss issues about work outside work. Perhaps if you contacted a member of Mrs Jones' family, they could help you with more information'. People will understand that you can't break confidentiality and perhaps will recognise that you would display the same regard for their privacy and respect you for it.

Case Study 2: You could leave the folder where it is for the nurse to come back to; after all, she left it there. However, this is breaching confidentiality regulations. The best thing to do would be to get the folder, find the nurse and let her know she left it on the bed. It is up to her then to keep it with her.

Case Study 3: This situation could escalate hugely if not dealt with correctly. The two staff members looking after Mr Armstrong have broken confidentiality regulations by discussing a client with someone who doesn't need to know anything about him. Not only that but they are discussing a client's personal issues in a public location, which is completely irrelevant to the care he is receiving. The family member could put in a serious complaint about the nurses to the point where disciplinary action could be taken.

Can you think of any other solutions in these scenarios?

Ways of Maintaining Confidentiality

+ Don't ever talk about your clients with your friends or family after your shift, however much you might want to.

+ Don't leave medical or nursing notes lying around.

+ Don't discuss clients with other clients.

+ Don't talk about clients with family members of other clients.

+ Don't discuss your clients with their family without their knowledge and (preferably) written consent.

+ Be conscious of a client's name being on display where it can be seen by the general public unless it is their room e.g. in a nursing home and the person has consented to it.

+ Be aware of talking loudly about clients in corridors or in open spaces where anyone can hear.

+ Don't give your computer password to someone else to use.

+ Don't give client information over the phone (unless there is a policy in place for doing so, in which case you must follow that policy to the letter).

+ Do be mindful of the person you are taking care of and respect them as a person.

+ Don't promise you will keep a secret when you are obliged to disclose a safeguarding issue e.g. suspected child/elder/domestic abuse.

+ Make sure you treat your client as you would like to be treated – would you want everyone to know your business?

+ Keep records safe and locked away if necessary.

+ Make sure that your computer is password protected when not in use.

+ Only discuss a client's condition with staff members who need to know.

+ Respect people's property e.g. letters, and make sure it is kept safe.

+ Do not discuss clinical information with relatives/visitors/friends and other residents – this is a nurse's duty and you should politely refer to the nurse in charge of the shift.

Clients' Belongings

Most people who enter healthcare settings will have some personal belongings with them. These can include items such as:

+ Handbags

+ Purse/wallets

+ Money

+ Mobile phones

+ Laptop/electronic devices

+ Clothing

+ Toiletries

+ Jewellery

+ Photographs and other personal effects.

Personal belongings can be invaluable to people. What may seem insignificant to you may hold cherished memories and meaning for someone.

Task **Stop and think!**
Think about your own belongings. What do they mean to you?

As a care worker you must remember to treat other people's property with the utmost care and respect. You must never go through or handle a person's property without their consent. If they are unable to give consent e.g. if they have dementia or if they are unconscious, then you must gain consent from their next of kin (NOK). If there is no NOK, then you must handle the property with care and ideally with another member of staff present to avoid any possible misunderstanding later. Obtaining consent shows that you respect your client.

Each healthcare setting will, or should, have their own policy concerning personal belongings.

Valuable Belongings Policy Example

Date Issued:	Review Date:	Title: Valuables Policy
Written/Reviewed by: Director of Nursing	Approved by:	Title:

1.0 Purpose: To provide clear guidelines about handling residents valuables and property

2.0. Scope: All Staff

3.0. Responsibilities: All Staff

4.0. Policy Statement:

4.1. This procedure must be followed by all staff when a resident is admitted to ******** Nursing Home.

4.2. All staff must respect resident's property.

4.3. All residents' property and valuables must be kept safe.

4.4. When a resident is admitted to ********* Nursing Home, a property list must be completed. The form must be dated and signed by either:

o   The resident and one member of staff who must also print their name and designation.

o   Two members of staff who must also print their name and designation.

o   Where the resident is unable to sign, a relative or Next of Kin (NOK) and a member of staff must sign.

4.4.1. Information about the resident's property must be clearly described e.g. 1 yellow jumper, 2 green cardigans etc.

4.4.2. Jewellery must be described in the following ways:

o   Silver must be written as 'white metal'.

o   Gold must be written as 'yellow metal'.

o   Any stones must be described by their colour e.g. diamond – clear stone; emerald – green stone; ruby – red stone etc.

4.5. Secure facilities must be provided for the safekeeping of money and valuables of the resident; ********** Nursing Home provides individual lockers with locks and keys for each bedroom. A locked safe is also available in the main office for those residents who wish to store valuables.

4.6. If the resident wishes to retain cash and/or valuables, they should be informed that ********* Nursing Home cannot be held responsible for cash and valuables retained by them.

4.6.1. They must sign an indemnity form.

4.6.2. It must be documented in the resident's notes/property list or care plan that they wish to retain the cash/valuables and have signed an indemnity form.

4.7. Residents will be advised to surrender large amounts of money or other valuables for safekeeping in the locked safe in the office.

4.8. A receipt book detailing the cash and valuables deposited into the safe will be maintained; this will be signed by whoever is putting the cash into the safe and witnessed by a second person. A copy of the details will be given to the resident for safekeeping.

4.9. Any cash or valuables taken out of the safe by the resident (or anyone on their behalf) must be signed for in the receipt book and written in the copy book.

4.10. A copy book will also be kept listing all properties kept within the safe.

This policy will be reviewed annually.

Signed: _____ **(Director of Nursing)**

Date: _____

(*Source:* With permission from the director of nursing, Shannon Lodge Nursing Home, Rooskey, Co. Roscommon.)

The policy clearly outlines the steps to be taken by staff in order to protect clients' property. The manager is responsible for ensuring that all his/her care workers are aware of and understand the policy. Care workers are required and have responsibility to familiarise themselves with the policy, making sure that they really do understand it. The policy should describe the process for checking property of a client on admission. This is part of the admission procedure that carers will be involved in.

Usually two staff members check property and fill out a property list describing the clothing and other belongings the client has bought in. Nursing homes will make sure that all clothes are labelled with name tags so clothes don't go missing if, for example, they are sent to the laundry as opposed to being taken by a relative to be washed at home.

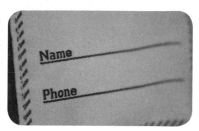

The system in hospitals may vary according to each ward and department. Residents and clients should be advised not to keep large amounts of money or valuable items. Instead they should be encouraged to let a trusted relative take it home for safekeeping or allow it to be placed in a safe where a record of its lodgement is made and a receipt given. To avoid any possible future misunderstanding, a record of all money and valuables taken home by a relative should be kept in the resident's/client's personal file.

Remember

+ Always treat people's property with the utmost respect and handle with care.

+ Think about how you would like your belongings to be handled.

+ Know your workplace policies and procedures in relation to personal belongings.

+ Make sure you fill out property lists correctly.

The Impact of Dependency on Clients and Carers

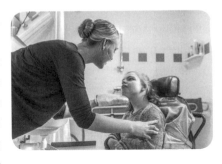

Before we start to think about what dependency means, let us reflect for a minute: did you need any help to get out of bed this morning? Help to have a wash? Did you need assistance whilst you ate your breakfast? Could you walk between each room getting whatever it was you needed? Did you choose what you were going to wear? Did you decide what time you were going to get out of bed? In fact, did you need any help at all?

Sometimes we take for granted that we can carry out these everyday tasks independently and make decisions for ourselves. Simple decisions and acts such as making a cup of tea can be completed on our own without including anyone else. Now imagine being dependent on someone else to help us with those everyday tasks: waiting for someone to come and get you up in the morning, to wash and dress you, to assist with mealtimes or to take you to the toilet. How would that be for you?

We are of course dependent on things such as money, friendship, love, shelter, food, oxygen, transport, water, but some of these are for survival and some are to enhance our quality of life. A definition of what it is to be dependent is as follows:

> Dependent, of or pertaining to a condition of being reliant on someone or something else for help, support, favour, and other needs, as a child is dependent on a parent, a narcotics addict is dependent on a drug, or one variable is dependent on another variable.
>
> (Anderson et al. 1994)

The opposite of dependence is, of course, independence. When we are independent, we can look after ourselves and meet our own needs. However, if we become dependent on something or someone, due for example to infirmity or general ill health, our lives can be totally changed. It can mean having to rely on someone else to meet our physical, social, spiritual or psychological needs and sometimes it might be a combination of all these needs (Nifast 2013). Being dependent on someone else can mean needing practical care and help with our Activities of Daily Living (ADLs) including:

✚ Washing and dressing

✚ Grooming – shaving, hair brushing, putting on make-up, cleaning teeth

✚ Eating and drinking

✚ Mobilising e.g. walking, getting into and out of a chair etc.

✚ Getting to and using the toilet.

It is very important for healthcare staff to help clients to be as independent as possible. An example of this would be to encourage the use of equipment such as walking aids to assist with mobility e.g. frames, sticks, rollators, wheelchairs etc.

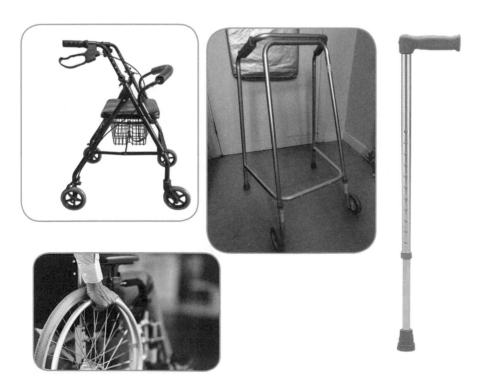

Encouraging independence can empower the client, improve self-esteem and the feeling of self-worth. Clients are individuals with varying care needs. Their level of dependency will be determined by several factors including their physical and mental health condition and even temporary illness. An individual assessment of their needs is necessary in order to ascertain their level of dependency and, therefore, the level of care required to meet those needs (Nifast 2013).

The level of care could include the number of carers required and the type of equipment needed. Dependency levels can be identified using varying assessment tools such as the 12 Activities of Daily Living by Roper, Logan and Tierney. This model is used to assess the level of dependency.

The 12 Activities of Daily Living (ADLs)

As mentioned above, one method of determining a person's level of dependency is the 12 Activities of Daily Living (Roper, Logan and Tierney 1996). An individual would be assessed against each of the activities to see if they require: no help; a little help; more than a little help; or full assistance with all the activities of daily living. The Activities of Daily Living (ADLs) are:

1. Maintaining a safe environment
2. Breathing
3. Eating and drinking
4. Washing and dressing
5. Communication
6. Mobilisation
7. Expressing sexuality
8. Controlling body temperature
9. Elimination
10. Working and playing
11. Sleeping
12. Dying

(Refer to page 117 for more detail on ADLs)

Being Dependent on Care

How must it feel to be dependent/reliant on someone to give you care? As carers we must recognise that clients who depend on us for their care needs may have the following feelings/emotions:

- **Vulnerability:** Feeling unsafe in, or unsure of, their new situation

- **Powerlessness:**
  - Feeling as though they are losing, or have lost, control of events

  - Struggling to adjust to the changes forced upon them through no fault of their own

  - Feeling as if they can't do anything about the situation they find themselves in

- **Worthlessness:**
  - Feeling as if they are of no use to themselves or anyone else

  - Feeling as if they are a burden to relatives and friends and even the carers who look after them.

Case Study: Being cared for – Gladys

I'm 86 and have lived in Sunnydale Nursing Home for the past five years. They look after me well here. I need help with washing and dressing in the morning and going to bed at night. I have a frame I walk with; it's a nuisance but it stops me from falling over. I must wait for a carer to walk with me. It's a bit annoying having to wait before I can get up. I've got used to asking for help now. I didn't like it at first because I was so independent when I was living in my own home. I used to bake, cook, clean and even drove my own car up until I was 80; but then I started having falls and my memory started to fail so I was 'advised' to stop driving. That was tough! Now if I want to go anywhere or do anything like have a cup of tea or a slice of cake, I need to ask someone. I think the hardest thing for me is being helped to the toilet, that can be very embarrassing. I never thought I'd see the day! I feel like a burden at times. The staff never complain but I feel like I'm nothing really, what's the point? I just sit here waiting for someone to come and get me. Still, I do enjoy going down for the movie on a Friday afternoon – but I must wait for one of the carers to come and get me and hope they come before the movie starts!

Task **Stop and think!**
As a HCA, if you were looking after Gladys how could you
encourage her to be independent and give her a sense of
self-worth?

Of course, on the other side of things is the carer. Some people will make
the big decision and commitment to look after a family member, a friend or
a neighbour who has become less able or totally unable to look after him or
herself. As a care worker you may work in 'home care' where you will be
going into people's own home and meeting family members/friends who
are 'carers'. They may have decided to take care of an individual for several
reasons without entirely realising what will be involved. At times they may
need some help and be glad to receive it. Looking after someone at home
can cause mixed emotions depending on the person's physical or mental
condition, how long the situation has been going on, family dynamics, living
arrangements and other things that might cause stresses and strains.

Case Study: Being a carer – Linda

I've looked after my mam for two years now. She was diagnosed
with vascular dementia three years ago. She coped in her own
home for the first year, but then a neighbour found her outside
down the road in her nightie, front door wide open. My sister and
I decided that she should move in with one of us. Dad died eight
years ago. Since then Mam's lived alone. They were close; life for
Mam has not been the same since he died. I work part-time and my
children are older than my sister's, so I said I'd look after Mam. I'm
happy to have her here where she's safe and content.

We've adapted the downstairs room for her and there is a shower
room and toilet so it's like she has her own living area. I'm not
saying it's easy, it's hard when she forgets who I am and she can
get cross. I bite my tongue and remember she's not well.

We say, 'She's our mammy and we have to take the rough with the smooth'. Mam bought up four of us and has six grandchildren, the least we can do is mind her. My sister is good and has Mam at the weekend so I can get a break. However, we are finding that it is becoming more confusing for Mam when she comes back so we are thinking we might have to stop this. We have carers in to help her wash in the morning, but I help her to bed in the evenings. It is tiring, especially when she gets up in the night. I don't like leaving her when I go to work. I worry that she might fall or injure herself even though we've done everything we can to make everywhere is as safe as possible. I'm scared for the future and whether she'll have to go to a nursing home. But for now I'm not thinking of that, we'll do what we can with what we have.

Task **Stop and think!**
If you were a HCA going into Linda's home to look after her mother, what could you do to help and support her mother, Linda and the family?

Even the best, the most professional and compassionate of carers may experience several emotions. These may include:

+ Ambivalence
+ Grief
+ Anxiety
+ Feeling under-appreciated
+ Boredom
+ Resentment

+ Crankiness, irritability
+ Anger
+ Depression
+ Impatience
+ Embarrassment
+ Fear

+ Disgust
+ Loneliness
+ Guilt
+ Tiredness
+ Jealousy
+ Loss

(*Source:* Family Caregiver Alliance, 2014)

A carer experiencing any of the above emotions should not feel guilty as these can be perfectly normal emotions. They might indicate that carers may need extra support and help.

As a caregiver, being aware that sometimes you may be the first person the family member sees in the morning is very important. They may have had a bad night with their loved one and so may be tired and irritable and may snap at you. You must not take this personally as they don't really mean to take it out on you. However, make sure you talk to your supervisor or manager and let them know what is happening. They may decide that it is necessary to talk to the family member. Caring for their loved one at home might be becoming too much and they may need to start thinking about residential/nursing home care. This can be a very difficult decision and needs to be handled sensitively. It is not your responsibility to become involved in this decision so you must hand this over to your supervisor.

Remember

+ Consider how it feels to be independent, to be able to make choices and decisions.

+ Consider how it would feel to be dependent on another person for your care needs.

+ There are dependency assessment tools to identify the dependency level of an individual in order to plan and implement care.

+ Always think about how your client may be feeling – be sympathetic, empathetic, kind and compassionate.

+ Consider how other family carers may be feeling.

+ Acknowledge that sometimes family members can be short with you, snap at you and criticise the care you are giving. Often this is because they are tired and feeling stressed. They will usually apologise.

> ✚ However, it is not acceptable for you to have to take verbal or physical abuse and you must make sure that you report all incidents to your supervisor and follow your company's policy regarding incident reports.

Essence of Care

The Five Concepts of Care

When you are caring for clients in healthcare settings, doing so in a kind, understanding, tender and sympathetic manner is so important. Do your best to show empathy or 'step into their shoes' and imagine how they may be feeling and think how you yourself would want to be cared for in the same circumstances. You should always remember what constitutes high-quality care. There are five main parts or aspects which are referred to as 'concepts'. These are:

1. Dignity
2. Privacy
3. Respect
4. Choice/Involvement
5. Autonomy/Independence.

These concepts are subjective, meaning that different people think of them in different ways and are therefore difficult to measure. They are interlinked with each other and, though slightly different, have very similar meanings.

Concept	Definition	The Concept in Practice
Dignity	The word, dignity, is derived from the Latin *dignus* meaning worthy. Being worthy or esteemed, being of high rank or position, or having a high opinion of oneself; self-esteem, stillness of manner; gravity (Mairis 1994; Allen 2001)	✛ The client feels valued, listened to, not belittled or made to feel worthless. ✛ Referred to by the name they wish to be called as opposed to a name you decide upon, or worse, a bed number ✛ Cared for in single-sex wards ✛ Given clean, fresh clothes ✛ If the client has had the misfortune to soil themselves and requires changing, cleaning them as quickly and as quietly as possible in a dignified and sympathetic manner.
Privacy	Freedom from intrusion Relates to all information and practice that is personal or sensitive in nature to an individual (UHB NHS Foundation Trust 2019)	✛ Pulling curtains around the bed ✛ Remembering that curtains are not walls and sounds will carry outside the cubicle ✛ Talking quietly but in a way that the client can easily hear ✛ Covering the client when carrying out personal care ✛ Being professional when handing over to colleagues and not being 'gossipy' ✛ Recognising that personal details are confidential and shouting personal information down the corridor is strictly not allowed

Concept	Definition	The Concept in Practice
Privacy *contd.*		✛ Speaking quietly in the rooms/ wards ✛ Ensuring that personal space is not being crowded by staff or visitors
Respect	Holding a person in high regard, valuing their opinion, recognising the client as a person (Beach et al. 2007)	✛ Gaining consent, approval or permission for your actions ✛ Calling the client by the name they wish to be called ✛ Introducing yourself and informing them who you are and why you are there ✛ Taking care in the way you speak and the words you use e.g. not using the words 'bib', 'nappy', 'toileting', 'feeding'. In other words, no 'baby' words or jargon ✛ Looking at the person to whom you are speaking and maintaining eye contact ✛ Not being overfriendly; being professional at all times ✛ Recognising people as individuals ✛ Providing information when appropriate and when asked (sometimes you might need to ask your manager) ✛ Showing empathy i.e. showing understanding about the person's situation ✛ Recognising and respecting different cultures and beliefs

Concept	Definition	The Concept in Practice
Choice/ Involvement	An act of choosing between two or more possibilities (Oxford English Dictionary)	+ Involving clients in their care plan and decisions about their future care + Providing choice about all aspects of care e.g. what food would they like and what they don't like; clothes they would like to wear
Autonomy/ Independence	Respecting people's capacity to make their own decisions and to control their own lives (Beauchamp and Childress 2013; Elcock et al. 2019)	+ Encouraging independence with ADLs e.g. washing and dressing + Recognising and treating the person as an individual and not just one of several clients + Providing information voluntarily and when requested + Encouraging the person to make their own decisions on a day-to-day basis and so help them understand that they are entitled to do so

Applying the Concepts of Care

As a care worker always remember that the client you care for in hospital, their own home, nursing home or outpatient clinic may feel vulnerable, frightened, in pain or nervous. They may never have been cared for before and will have to undergo the difficult process of being asked personal questions, being examined and asked to undress.

Some clients will have to be assisted with ADLs e.g. being taken to the toilet, being washed, dressed and assisted with mealtimes. In these circumstances a person will have difficulty in feeling dignified, so you will have to do everything possible to help them. Therefore, the care provided by you and the team must be carried out in a dignified, respectful, understanding, friendly and professional manner to make sure that a difficult experience becomes a more bearable one.

However, if a carer fails to show these characteristics, obviously the opposite can happen, with the result that the client has a traumatic experience and is left feeling worthless, dehumanised and undignified. It can even lead to safe-guarding issues. Therefore, it is so important that all HCAs are trained in and clearly understand how to apply the basic principles of the concepts of care when nursing clients in whatever care settings they are in. Your interactions will help to build the relationship to make people feel valued, at ease and confident in the care that they are receiving. For you, it is your job: you are used to the care environment, but clients are not. You need to be aware that everything you do when you deliver care will have an impact, good or bad, on the client; so, introduce yourself, tell them what your role is, ask them how they are feeling, and don't forget that a smile can make a world of difference.

#Hello My Name Is Campaign

Kate Granger was a doctor, but also a terminally ill cancer patient. During a hospital stay Kate observed that many

hello my name is…

staff looking after her did not introduce themselves before delivering care. She felt so strongly about the importance of this basic step in communication that she and her husband started a campaign using social media to encourage and remind healthcare staff about the importance of introductions. This campaign is called '#hellomynameis …'

Kate felt that introductions were about making a human connection between one human being who is suffering and vulnerable, and another who wishes to help. The first tweet Kate and her husband sent was '#hellomynameis is the first rung on the ladder to providing truly person-centred, compassionate care'. This campaign was a worldwide success and continues to be as relevant and important today.

(See: https://www.hellomynameis.org.uk/)

Task Activity
Practise 'Hello, my name is ...' with your class.

Case Study: Mrs Mahony

Two carers went into Mrs Mahony's room and said brightly 'Morning!' as they opened the curtains. They pulled back the bed covers and said that it was time to get up for breakfast and asked if Mrs Mahony had a good night's sleep. They helped her into the bathroom and onto the toilet, chatting about this and that and being friendly and kind. They helped Mrs Mahony back into the room, got her clothes that had been laid out the night before and, after washing her, helped her get dressed. Whilst they were dressing Mrs Mahony, another carer popped her head round the door to see if they needed any help. She cheerily said hello to Mrs Mahony but left quickly when the two carers said they were okay. Once all of Mrs Mahony's care needs were attended to, she was helped into a wheelchair and taken down to the dining room for her breakfast.

Task Stop and think!
What would you do differently?

Think about what happened in this scenario?

Was Mrs Mahony's dignity maintained?

Was her privacy and choice maintained and respect displayed?

Considerations: In this case study, although the carers were bright and friendly, we are unsure whether Mrs Mahony has met them before. The carers failed to introduce themselves to her, they opened the curtains in the room where she would be getting dressed, probably therefore not affording her any privacy. She doesn't appear to have been given any choice about getting out of bed or asked whether she would like to go to the toilet, have a wash or even what type of wash she would like to have. Mrs Mahony's clothes had been laid the night before, but we are not told if she had chosen to wear those clothes or if they had been chosen for her. The other carer did not appear to knock so failed to respect Mrs Mahony's privacy.

By failing to respect her dignity, choice and independence, Mrs Mahony was in some ways disempowered and not provided with the highest quality of care.

Dignity in Care Campaign

Launched in November 2006 in the UK, the Dignity in Care campaign aims to put dignity and respect at the heart of care services. The campaign's core values are about having dignity in hearts, minds and actions, changing the culture of services and placing a greater emphasis on improving the quality of care and the experience of clients.

The campaign developed a 10 Point Dignity Challenge (now called the 10 Dignity Do's) describing values and actions that high-quality services, who respect people's dignity, should strive towards:

1. Have a zero tolerance of all forms of abuse

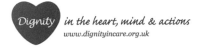
Dignity in the heart, mind & actions
www.dignityincare.org.uk

2. Support people with the same respect you would want for yourself or a member of your family

3. Treat each person as an individual by offering a personalised service

4. Enable people to maintain the maximum possible level of independence, choice and control

5. Listen and support people to express their needs and wants

6. Respect people's right to privacy

7. Ensure people feel able to complain without fear of retribution

8. Engage with family members and carers as care partners

9. Assist people to maintain confidence and positive self-esteem

10. Act to alleviate people's loneliness and isolation

(*Source:* https://www.dignityincare.org.uk/About/Dignity_in_Care_campaign/)

Case Study: Ms Farrell

A 30-year-old woman, Ms Farrell, having suffered a miscarriage at eleven weeks, is taken into the A&E department in which you are working. In a wheelchair, she is taken into the cubicle area by a porter, but because she is feeling faint, she is helped onto a trolley and left in the cubicle alone with no blanket to cover her.

Task

Stop and think!

How do you think Ms Farrell felt before she had even been seen by medical staff?

Was her dignity maintained?

How could she have been comforted?

Case Study: Mr James Carling

A 55-year-old homeless man, Mr James Carling, is admitted to a medical ward. He is wearing a gown and is very dishevelled. On admission, two carers, a male and female, introduce themselves to the man and ask him what he would like to be called. He says that they can call him Jim. They offer to give him a shower, which he accepts. They get fresh pyjamas for him, towels and toiletries. They tell him all about the ward he is on, explain about the food, who works on the ward and how he can ask for help whenever he needs it. They show him the call bell. They explain how the clothes he was wearing can be sent to be laundered if he wants and that he can wear the hospital pyjamas until they can get fresh clothes for him. They then help Jim to the shower room where they close the door. They then help him with the shower but letting and encouraging him to do as much as he can himself. When they help him to dry himself, they cover him with a towel so that he is not exposed. He has a shave and brushes his hair. He looks like a new man! Once he is clean and fresh, they assist him back to bed and make sure he is comfortable. They again show him where his call bell is and make sure he is safe.

Task **Stop and think!**
How do you think the five elements in the Essence of Care have been adhered to in the case of Jim?

Design and Dignity Programme – The Irish Hospice Foundation

The Design and Dignity Programme initiated by the Irish Hospice Foundation is grounded in the firm belief that the end of life should be recognised as a time of the most intense human feelings, which can include sadness, loss, anxiety and fear. These feelings should not have to be endured in inappropriate surroundings: a busy corridor, a waiting room, a ward, a reception area – places where others may be chatting and laughing.

The Irish Hospice Foundation is working to renovate areas such as shabby storage rooms to turn them into oases of calm where bad news can be broken sensitively or where families can gather and have a cup of tea. They are redesigning viewing rooms where people first see a deceased loved one, with quiet anterooms provide families and loved ones with a space where they can compose themselves. They are transforming neglected mortuaries into havens of peace. (See https://hospicefoundation.ie/design-dignity/)

'Our vision is that there will be end-of-life sanctuaries in every adult, paediatric and maternity hospital in Ireland, designed to ensure that death and dying are experienced in surroundings that enhance dignity and respect for patients and for their families.'

End-of-life sanctuaries include palliative care suites for patients who are dying, family rooms with overnight accommodation, counselling rooms for bereaved families, bereavement suites in emergency department units and family-friendly mortuaries.

(*Source:* https://hospicefoundation.ie/design-dignity/)

chapter 10

PLANNING FOR AND MEETING CLIENT NEEDS

IN THIS CHAPTER YOU WILL LEARN ABOUT:

+ Understanding the care needs of clients throughout their lifespan

+ Person-centred care and care planning

+ The concept of individuality

+ Cultural awareness

The Care Needs of Clients throughout Their Lifespan

People may have different care needs throughout their lifespan. Care needs are those required by a client to achieve and maintain their best level of physical health and a feeling of being within their circumstances. This also includes their psychological and spiritual wellbeing. Clients will require different kinds of assistance and support with different care needs. As healthcare professionals it is your role to support and encourage them to achieve their best potential physical and mental health (Nifast 2013).

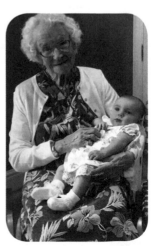

101-year-old great-grandmother with her three-month-old great-granddaughter

Clients' care needs can be assessed using the holistic approach which has been defined as follows:

'The holistic concept places the client/resident at the centre of care and recognises that each individual is unique and must be viewed from the perspective of the physical, emotional, social, psychological and spiritual needs' (Goodwin Chew 2011).

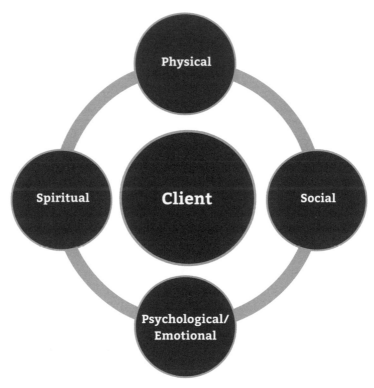

Physical Needs

- Washing and dressing
- Toilet requirements
- Safe environment, accident free
- Nutrition needs (food and fluid)
- Rest and sleep
- Exercise
- Level of dependence
- Relief of pain/distress
- Change of position/ pressure sore prevention.

Psychological/Emotional Needs

+ Being listened to
+ Being understood
+ Polite and respectful communication
+ Having feelings acknowledged
+ Person-centred care
+ Autonomy
+ Feeling safe and secure in your own home

+ Respect and understanding of beliefs, values, culture, needs and wishes without being judged
+ Feeling part of your own family
+ Privacy
+ Dignity.

Social Needs

+ Social interaction
+ Relatives/visitors
+ Activities/community organisations/support organisations
+ Employment/work opportunities

+ Likes/dislikes
+ Home life etc.
+ Friends and family
+ What we like doing for enjoyment.

Spiritual Needs

+ Beliefs
+ Respect and acceptance of religion and cultural customs
+ Access to a minister/priest or other religious and cultural advisors

+ Death beliefs and customs
+ Prayer rituals
+ Special foods.

Task **Stop and think!**
Using this holistic model, think of as many care needs as possible that a client may have.

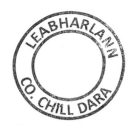

The Hierarchy of Needs

The humanist theorist Abraham Maslow (1908–1970) explained that a person has basic needs that must be met for a person to survive, function and to ultimately be all they can be (O'Brien 2013).

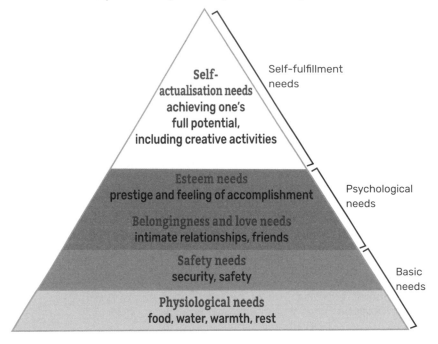

Maslow created a five-tier model of human needs called the Hierarchy of Needs beginning with basic physiological needs, moving through to more complex psychological needs such as security and esteem. Maslow identified that the needs listed at one level must be at least partially satisfied before moving onto the next level (O'Brien 2013). For example, while we all recognise that safety is important, it is almost irrelevant if the need for oxygen, food and drink is not met. This principle and approach underline and identify what the basic human needs are and also what motivates people.

Physiological needs	Oxygen, food, water, clothing, sex, sleep
Safety needs	Security, feeling safe from harm or danger
	Safe environment
	Financial security

Love and belonging	Love, closeness, affection, family, friends
Esteem needs	To think well of oneself, and to see oneself as useful and having value
	People often lack self-esteem when ill, injured, older or disabled
Self-actualisation needs	Achieving one's own potential
	Involves learning, understanding and creating to the limit of a person's capacity
	The highest need, rarely totally met
	This need can be postponed, and life will continue.

As healthcare workers, the model can be applied in practice to ensure needs are being met. Not only should we be providing food and water for clients, we should also be keeping them safe and free from harm whilst empowering them to do as much as possible for themselves and giving them a sense of belonging. A way of doing this is by adopting a person-centred approach to care.

Person-Centred Care and Care Planning

Person-centred care is an approach to nursing and social care work that puts the client at the centre of the decision-making process about their health and care needs (Elcock et al. 2019). The term 'person-centred' may also be referred to as:

+ Individualised care

+ Personalised care

+ Patient-centred care

+ Client-centred care.

(*Source:* RCNI 2016; Hindle and Coates 2011)

In the past, care and treatment were decided by doctors and nurses without any input from clients or family. This approach could have been deemed as being disempowering for the client, resulting in a lack of control and diminishing their dignity (Elcock et al. 2019).

The person-centred approach aims to do the opposite. It empowers the client to be in control of their care, to be involved in the care planning process and to have a voice that should be listened to. It is an approach whereby the MDT takes into consideration the views and wishes of the client, their values and beliefs. There may be disagreements about the plan of care and treatment, but with good teamwork, positive communication and discussion an effective plan can be created.

The nurse's role when first seeing a client is to use the holistic approach along with other assessment tools to assess the client's varying needs and personal preferences. The assessment and care planning process would be carried out alongside the client and often close family members would be involved too.

As a member of the MDT, the HCA would be aware of the individual care plan that has been created for the client and will work alongside the nurse to deliver it.

The Process of Care Planning

When a client is admitted to a care facility they will need to be assessed and a plan of care written for them. To begin with, the nurse or whoever is carrying out the assessment will use an assessment tool, usually the Nursing Process, the steps of which are:

+ Assessment
+ Nursing diagnosis
+ Planning
+ Implementation
+ Evaluation.

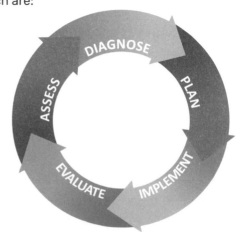

The 12 Activities of Daily Living

Along with the nursing process, the nurse will also use the holistic approach to identify the physical, psychological, spiritual and social needs of the client.

A nursing model is also used to assess the needs, the most common one being Roper, Logan and Tierney's 12 Activities of Daily Living (ADLs).

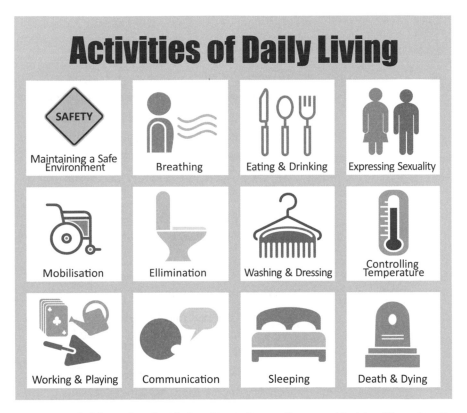

The **12 Activities of Daily Living (ADLs)** are often used to identify a client's actual or potential problems.

✦ **Actual problems:** Require addressing immediately – an example would be a low blood sugar level, in which case a client would need treatment immediately, before it became worse.

✦ **Potential problems:** Complications could occur so preventative measures are put in place to stop the potential problem from becoming an actual one. For example, a client with a high Waterlow

Score (tool to assess the likelihood of a client developing a pressure sore) would be nursed in a bed with a pressure-relieving mattress in place to prevent the formation of pressure sores.

Listed below are the 12 ADLs and examples of observations/questions the nurse may use when assessing the client. This gives an idea of how much detail goes into an assessment (Roper, Logan and Tierney 1996).

ADL	Observations made/questions that may be asked
1. Maintaining a safe environment	+ Age of client + Do they live alone? + Do they have any conditions such as dementia, Alzheimer's? + What is their knowledge of and attitude to maintaining a safe environment? + Are they aware of fire safety, accidents, fall risks? + Have they had any difficulties in the past in this area, and if so, how have these been coped with? + Can they walk; do they have an unsteady gait? Do they have a walking aid? + Are there environmental obstacles to mobility such as uneven floors, stairs, unsuitable footwear? + Other considerations: free from abuse, sensory deprivation, psychological and emotional wellbeing
2. Breathing	+ Does the client have any conditions such as asthma or Chronic Obstructive Pulmonary Disease (COPD) that can affect breathing? + Do they have any current problems with breathing? + Have they had any past problems or long-standing difficulties with breathing? If so, how have they coped?

ADL	Observations made/questions that may be asked
2. **Breathing** *contd.*	+ Could they potentially have any future problems? + Other considerations: do they smoke? How far can they walk without becoming breathless? Are there signs of cyanosis (blueness around lips or fingertips)? Do they need oxygen? Do they have inhalers/nebulisers? Does it help them to sit in certain positions?
3. **Eating and drinking**	+ Does the client have any conditions such as diabetes, coeliac disease, dysphagia? + How, what and when do they usually eat and drink? + Do they have any long-term problems with eating and drinking? If so, how have they been dealt with? + Other considerations: weight loss/gain, state of mouth and teeth, swallowing, appetite, modified diet, thickened fluid, alternative ways of assisting at mealtimes, PEG tube/NG tube
4. **Expressing sexuality**	+ Tip! Be sensitive in this area, don't make assumptions, be respectful. Some people will find this area very uncomfortable to discuss. + Does the client have any long-standing problems with expressing sexuality? + Are there any current problems in this area? If so, how have they coped? + Are any problems likely to develop? + Other considerations: identity/orientation, sexually transmitted disease, sexual development, sexual abuse, body image issues and fertility

ADL	Observations made/questions that may be asked
5. Mobilising	+ Does the client have any conditions affecting mobility such as amputation, stroke, dementia, motor neurone disease, post-surgery, multiple sclerosis, osteoporosis, broken bones?
	+ What age is the client? (infancy – increasing skills; adolescence and adulthood – peak performance; later years – less agile)
	+ Can they walk unaided, are they unsteady?
	+ Do they require a walking aid?
	+ Do they get much exercise?
	+ Do they have any current problems in this area? If so, how have they coped?
	+ Are any problems likely to develop?
	+ Other considerations: risk of falls, housing conditions (e.g. stairs), attitude towards safety and exercise, dependency level
6. Elimination – toilet needs	+ Tip! Incontinence, stoma bags etc. can cause embarrassment to clients. Be sensitive in this area, don't make assumptions, be respectful. Some people will find this area very uncomfortable to discuss.
	+ How often and when does the client eliminate urine/faeces?
	+ Are there any factors that impact the process of eliminating urine/faeces?
	+ Are there any current problems in this area? If so, how have they coped?
	+ What problems are likely to develop?
	+ Other things to consider: self-caring when going to the toilet, functioning urinary and defecatory systems, embarrassment, privacy and dignity, continence aids

ADL	Observations made/questions that may be asked
7. **Washing and dressing**	✛ Does the client have any conditions affecting washing and dressing such as stroke, dementia, Chronic Obstructive Pulmonary Disease (COPD)? ✛ What is their usual washing and dressing habit or routine? ✛ When and how often are they performed? ✛ What factors influence washing and dressing? ✛ Are there any long-standing difficulties? ✛ Are there any current problems in this area? If so, how have they coped? ✛ Other things to consider: religious and cultural requirements, age, observation of skin, hair, nails, teeth, emotional state, dignity and privacy, likes and dislikes regarding showers baths
8. **Controlling body temperature**	✛ Does the client find their body temperature to be too high, too low or comfortable? ✛ How do they control their own body temperature? ✛ Are there any potential risks in relation to hyper or hypothermia? ✛ Are there any current problems in this area? If so, how have they coped? ✛ Other things to consider: exercise, hormones, time of day, age, gender, environment, pregnancy, menopause
9. **Working and playing**	✛ Tip! Long-term chronic illness can affect this activity of living. Finding out the client's job/hobbies can be significant in relation to their illness. Have they inhaled dust or fumes, for example?

ADL	Observations made/questions that may be asked
9. **Working and playing** *contd.*	+ How much time do they spend in work/play and when?
	+ Are there any current problems in this area? If so, how have they coped?
	+ Could there be any potential problems in this area?
	+ Other things to consider: sometimes work and leisure life must be adapted due to ill health e.g. someone whose mobility has been affected may have to change their hobby from running to swimming. Encouraging people to get involved in exercise can help reduce mental health problems and depression
10. **Communicating**	+ Does the client have any conditions affecting communication such as stroke, dementia, motor neurone disease?
	+ Are there any potentially relevant factors in relation to their age, development or life experience that may affect communication style?
	+ Do they normally need any kind of help to communicate and interact with others in either one-to-one or group situations?
	+ Do they have a preferred means of communication?
	+ Does the care setting have the means to meet normal communication needs?
	+ What family/friend support network does the client normally have?
	+ What problems, if any, does the person have at present with communicating, or seem likely to develop?
	+ Other things to consider: self-confidence, hearing, vision, reading, writing, gestures, tone, listening, body language, eye contact

ADL	Observations made/questions that may be asked
11. Sleeping	+ Does the client have any conditions affecting sleeping such as sleep apnoea, insomnia, stress and anxiety?
	+ What is their age (people of different ages need different amounts of sleep)?
	+ What are their normal sleeping patterns?
	+ Do they take anything to help them sleep (natural or prescription)?
	+ How many hours do they normally sleep for?
	+ What time do they wake?
	+ Does anything affect their sleeping pattern?
	+ Other things to consider: environmental factors; does the person sleep with a light on, window open; is there overcrowding where they live? Homelessness, shift work, what do they do before they go to sleep? What helps them to relax?
12. Dying	+ The assessment will depend upon the client's circumstances. If it is end-of-life care, the care plan will be very detailed in this area.
	+ What is the age of the client?
	+ What do they (and their family) know about the condition and length of time they have left to live?
	+ What are their beliefs about dying and death?
	+ What affect will the dying process have on them and their family?
	+ Are they and their family going through the grieving process?
	+ What are their religious and cultural requirements?

ADL	Observations made/questions that may be asked
12. Dying *contd.*	✚ What do they and their family want the healthcare worker to do when the death occurs? ✚ Other things to consider: care of the family, practical care of the client, fears, anxieties and feelings, multidisciplinary approach

(*Source:* Roper, Logan and Tierney, 1996)

Once the client's needs have been identified the nurse can write an individualised care plan. It is becoming increasingly common for care facilities to have computerised care plans and other records. Care plans should be reviewed and evaluated regularly as required and especially if circumstances change.

The assessment is carried out by doing the following:

✚ Talking to the client and their family

✚ Listening to them

✚ Using observational skills – looking at the client, colour of skin, monitoring urine and bowel movements etc.

✚ Taking vital signs – blood pressure, pulse, respiration rate, oxygen saturation, temperature

✚ Reading medical notes.

The role of the nurse is to carry out the assessment and formulate the care plan. However, the role of the HCA is to help the nurse implement that care. It is important for HCAs to have knowledge of the assessment and care planning process so they can report any changes they may observe immediately to the person in charge. This can make a huge difference to a client and can stop a potential problem from becoming an actual one.

Task **Stop and think!**
Read the two case studies that follow and think about what you would do in each scenario.

Case Study: **Jo and Minnie**

It is a busy morning on Ward 6 and Jo is helping Minnie to have a wash and change into a new nightie. As Jo is changing Minnie, she touches her skin and thinks to herself that Minnie feels very warm.

What should Jo do?

Case Study: **Sarah**

Sarah James is 82 years old. Sarah is a widow; she has four children and six grandchildren. She has been admitted to a nursing home following discharge from hospital. She had a stroke four weeks previously and has been receiving treatment since. She has a right-sided weakness and slurred speech. She has good eyesight, but is unable to hear well without the use of a hearing aid. She also needs assistance with mobilisation. Occasionally Sarah is incontinent of urine. She requires thickened fluids and a pureed diet due to poor swallowing function. She also has arthritis and has pain in her joints, particularly on movement. Sarah used to be involved in the local church and enjoys reading and seeing her friends and family. She has expressed how nervous she is about the future and about living in a nursing home.

Using the 12 ADLs, identify Sarah's actual and potential problems. Remember: actual problems are problems that need to be dealt with immediately (priority problems) and potential problems are problems that are anticipated/problems that might happen.

Identity and Individuality

"Who in the world am I?" Ah, that's the great puzzle.

From Alice's Adventures in Wonderland *by Lewis Carroll*

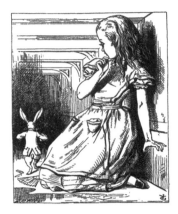

Alice asks this question of herself after she grows to a giant size. Alice is not only trying to make sense of the surreal surroundings of Wonderland but also of her own identity and changing sense of self (Aihong 2014).

We might often feel like Alice, asking ourselves the same sort of questions. Who are we? Where do we fit in? What is our role?

The *Penguin Concise English Dictionary* defines 'identity' as:

> Who or what somebody or something is. The individual characteristics that define a person or thing or by which a person or thing can be recognised. The condition of being exactly alike; sameness.
>
> (Allen 2001)

Our identity is important to us, it makes us who we are. It gives us a sense of meaning and belonging. Our name is part of our identity. We can be identified by our Personal Public Service (PPS) number, passport, fingerprint (we all have unique fingerprints) and by our dental records.

Task **Stop and think!**
Think about your identity: what makes you, you?

How would you describe yourself?

Our identity can be shaped by the following:

✦ **Physical appearance:** This is often the first thing to be seen that identifies a person: height, weight, the man with a moustache and tattoos, the lady with the glasses and long hair. When we change our physical appearance, people notice; 'Have you changed your hairstyle?' We like to be noticed and love to be asked, 'Have you had your hair done?' or 'Have you got new glasses?' The clothes we wear can say a lot about us. We may wear a uniform which would tell people about our job, or maybe a football kit, or a jacket for a running club which would shout out that we belonged to that club.

✦ **Gender:** Some people are content to identify themselves as the gender they were born into. However, for some it is less straightforward. For example, they may be born biologically male but identify themselves as female (trans woman). Some individuals may be uncertain about their identity and wish to be identified as both male and female (gender fluid) and some don't assign a gender identity at all (agender, genderless). Some choose to change their biological gender to match their gender identity by having surgery (gender reassignment) and taking hormones (Dustagheer et al. 2005; Neary and Cross 2018).

✦ **Sexuality:** Sexual orientation refers to physical, emotional and sexual attraction to another person. A person may be attracted to someone of the same gender (homosexual, gay or lesbian), they may be attracted to a person of the opposite gender (heterosexual), they may be attracted to both sexes (bisexual) or they may even be attracted to a person regardless of sex or gender (pansexual) (LGBT Ireland, 2018).

✦ **Religion:** Belonging to a religion e.g. Christianity, Buddhism etc. can give us a sense of identity. We may feel that we fit in with other people who have the same beliefs and have something in common. We may attend the same religious ceremonies, helping us to feel that we fit in.

+ **Race:** People born in other countries or to parents who were born in another country may identify differently to you. You will need to recognise and understand this.

+ **Culture and ethnicity:** People's identity is shaped by where they were born or brought up e.g. in another country. As a result they may be accustomed to different beliefs which might seem strange to you. You will need to recognise and understand this.

+ **Occupation:** Our occupation can define us; it can be our identity – people may be known as the 'nurse', the 'carer' or the 'social worker'. Often our occupation becomes part of who we are.

Each client has their own identity that makes them an individual. They may have many roles in their life, for example, a mother, father, brother, sister etc. Each person has a unique personality with a variety of characteristics, qualities and quirks that makes them an individual.

When caring for people we must be aware that people have different traits and this can affect the way they deal or cope with illness, difficult news, painful situations and being in vulnerable positions. Some people will make jokes whilst hiding their true feelings whereas others will openly talk about their feelings, wear their hearts on their sleeves, cry and maybe even shout.

We may carry out the same tasks with our clients e.g. bed bathing, taking observations, assisting someone with their food and drink, but we must never approach these in the same way. We must adopt an individualised approach remembering the core values of care: compassion, dignity, respect and empathy. So, when a person requires help with washing and dressing which are routine tasks, the individualised approach would be to consider their cultural needs, if they prefer a bath or shower, the type of shower gel/shampoo they like. The HCA needs to know the client's likes, dislikes and how they can be made to feel comfortable. If the client is treated as an individual as opposed to the same as everyone else, they will feel special, listened to, respected, cared for and an experience that may be an unpleasant one can be made much more bearable.

Case Study: Joe's individuality

Joe is being helped to have a shower by two carers. They are chatting with him nicely and kindly and he enjoys their company. In the bathroom there is a selection of his favourite shower gels and shampoo that his daughter Helen gave him for Christmas. They are on a high shelf and the carers don't see them. One of the carers goes and gets some shower gel from the trolley and uses that without asking Joe if he likes it. When they are helping Joe to get dressed, they can't find any trousers for him. Instead of going to the laundry room, they grab a spare pair from the trolley and one of the carers says, 'These will do for now until we find his own'.

Task **Stop and think!**

Do you think Joe is being treated as an individual here?

What could be done to improve the situation?

Case Study: Eliza's individuality

Eliza was admitted to Meadowhill Nursing Home for respite following a hip operation. The nurse on admission asked her what type of food she liked. When Eliza saw the menu, she said that she didn't like much of what was on offer and appeared disappointed. The nurse and a carer sat down with Eliza and worked out an individual menu for her. The food was ordered in and the kitchen staff made aware of Eliza's needs.

Task **Stop and think!**

What was the good practice here?

How do you think Eliza felt in this situation?

In the world of care, it is vital that we appreciate the uniqueness of each person that we care for; each with their own identity and individuality. If we don't have and show an understanding of this there could be a danger of appearing to be prejudiced and discriminatory. This might unintentionally result in the standard of care falling below what is expected and required, complaints and even possible safeguarding issues.

As carers, it is important to remember that even just the little things we do can make a huge difference to how someone feels. Things such as remembering someone's name, if they like tea or coffee or who their family members are will all help them to feel that they are being looked after by someone who really does care for them.

Diversity Awareness

> It is time for parents to teach young people early on that in diversity there is beauty and there is strength.
>
> (Maya Angelou 2014)

The population in Ireland is expanding and with this expansion there has been a significant growth in different cultures, religion and spiritual beliefs and lifestyles. People have moved from across the world for many different reasons to build new lives in Ireland. This movement of people brings significant diversities that can be challenging but need to be recognised, and, where appropriate, accepted and integrated into society. Diversity can mean many things: it can be a mixture, a variety or an assortment.

Task **Stop and think!**
List all the areas of diversity you can think of.

Some of the well-known areas of diversity include:

+ Lifestyle
+ Culture
+ Religion and spiritual beliefs
+ Race
+ Gender

+ Nationality
+ Sexual orientation
+ Age
+ Education
+ Occupation.

Healthcare professionals must recognise that diversity is all around us. They will work with colleagues and care for people who have different values, opinions and beliefs and these must be respected, even those that are not liked or agreed with. If we all had the same opinions and attitudes, the world would be a pretty boring place. Diversity adds interest.

Lifestyle

The **lifestyle** of a particular person or group of people is the living conditions, behaviour and habits that are typical of them or are chosen by them.

(https://www.collinsdictionary.com/dictionary/english/lifestyle)

Lifestyle is how a person lives their life. Of course, this can be affected by social, economic and environmental factors. These can include: the area a person lives in; who they live with; whether they have a social support network; accessibility of medical services; level of income; employment opportunities; type of housing and accessibility of transport. These factors are often out of our control however, but there are lifestyle choices that an individual can make that **are** controllable (Nifast 2013).

Lifestyle choices are 'decisions made by individuals about their consumptions of goods, services and culture' (Giddens 2001).

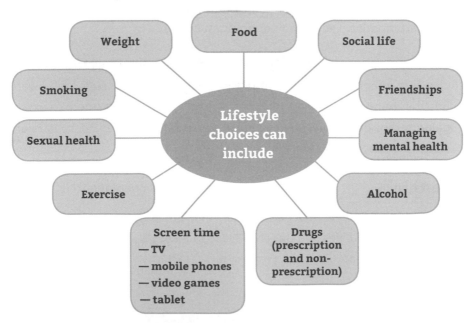

> **Task** **Stop and think!**
> List all your lifestyle choices.

The choice a person makes can lead to a positive or negative lifestyle. Poor or ill-judged lifestyle choices can have dire consequences on a person's health.

> **Task** **Stop and think!**
> Can you list some lifestyle choices that may affect health?

In Ireland over the last number of years there has been a drive towards healthy lifestyles. In 2004, for example, under the Public Health (Tobacco) Act, smoking in general workplaces was banned. This was a massive step towards encouraging people to stop smoking.

There has been a huge amount of work done in relation to mental health in the last several years. The HSE campaigns 'Little Things' and 'Mind Monsters' are two such examples of recent work to help people who suffer with mental health issues and show how such issues can affect their lifestyle (www.hse.ie). Other campaigns include 'Get Ireland Active', 'Healthy Eating', 'Health Promoting' and 'Schools and Drug Awareness'. (For more information, see www.healthpromotion.ie.)

Obviously as a HCA, promoting healthy choices without dictating to the client is important. Healthy lifestyles include getting sufficient sleep, healthy eating, not smoking, reducing alcohol intake, getting more exercise, being aware of and avoiding possible causes of diseases such as heart disease, diabetes and even dementia.

Culture

Census 2016 identified that 535,475 non-Irish nationals were living in Ireland coming from 200 different nations. These included people from Poland, UK, Lithuania, America, Germany, France, Italy and Romania (CSO.ie).

With this growth in migration comes significant diversity in culture, ethnicity and religion.

'Culture is commonly defined as the learned and shared values, beliefs, behaviours and customs of a group of people' (HSE 2009).

Task

Stop and think!
Think about your own culture – what are the common beliefs and values? What else influences a culture?

Culture can involve beliefs, values, behaviour and ways of life that are passed on from generation to generation. The beliefs, values and ways of life can include the following:

+ Language
+ Clothing
+ Food
+ Religion and spirituality
+ Traditions

+ Rituals
+ Etiquette
+ Lifestyle
+ Holidays.

(Carter and Goldschmidt 2010)

Examples of this in Ireland would be First Holy Communion which usually takes places in Second Class in many Catholic schools, or St Patrick's Day, 17 March, which is a national bank holiday and is celebrated widely throughout the country.

As Ireland becomes increasingly multicultural, it is crucial that all healthcare professionals are knowledgeable about cultural differences. An important part of the HCA role is to be aware of, and know something about, clients' ethnic backgrounds, in order to provide excellent quality care or to avoid offending the client or their family members, or both.

A recommendation made in the National Intercultural Health Strategy 2018–2023 was that staff will be provided with intercultural awareness training in order to 'ensure the provision of high-quality, culturally responsive services to service users from diverse ethnic, cultural and religious backgrounds' (HSE 2018b).

Education can be carried out within healthcare settings as in-house training or as part of education programmes such as the QQI courses.

Being culturally sensitive is vital. Sometimes we can be afraid to speak to people about their cultural needs for fear of saying the wrong thing or 'putting our foot in it'. So how can we be culturally sensitive?

Task **Stop and think!**
What does cultural sensitivity mean?

How can you be culturally sensitive in your place of work or whilst on work experience?

It is important to remember that everyone is an individual and therefore some clients may not feel or believe the same things about their culture as other people who belong to the same cultural group. Avoiding stereotyping or generalising is important. In order to be culturally sensitive some of the actions to take include:

+ Being polite

+ Being respectful in the way you speak

+ Being interested and learning about their culture

+ Asking open-ended questions about their cultural needs

+ Avoiding stereotyping and labelling

+ Being self-aware of your own cultural values and how these may cause prejudice or bias against the client's culture

+ Accepting people for who they are

+ If there are language barriers, finding alternative ways to communicate e.g. translators, family, pictures

+ Speaking to family and friends about cultural requirements

+ Attending training sessions about cultural awareness.

(Benson 2000; Nifast 2013)

Religion and Spirituality

Religion is accepted as 'the service and worship of God or the supernatural, commitment or devotion to religious faith or observance, a personal set or institutionalized system of religious attitudes, beliefs, and practices'.

(*Source:* https://www.merriam-webster.com/dictionary/religion)

In some religions people believe in a 'divine force' rather than personalised gods. In other religions, there are figures who are not gods, but who are thought of with reverence, for example the Buddha in Buddhism.

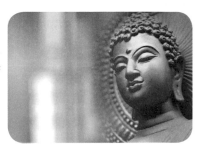

Ritual acts can include chanting, singing, praying, eating certain kinds of food or refraining from doing so, or fasting on certain days.

As with a client's cultural requirements, it is important to be aware of their religious and spiritual needs. On admission it should be established if a client has any religious or spiritual beliefs and how they wish for this to be catered for whilst being cared for.

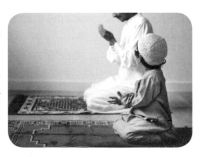

These beliefs/needs may include:

Dietary requirements	Clients' dietary requirements can be guided by their religious and cultural beliefs. For example, Muslims should be served Halal (lawful) food which has been ritually slaughtered. Muslim people do not eat pork and alcohol is prohibited.
	Devout Muslims may wish to fast during the month of Ramadan (no intake of food or drink between sunrise and sunset). A very sick Muslim is exempt from Ramadan.

Dietary requirements *contd.*	Jewish people are not allowed to eat any pig products. They may eat only Kosher meat which is a Jewish traditional way of slaughtering meat. Many Buddhists are vegetarians. (Benson 2000)
Religious/ spiritual practices	This can include worship, prayer, chanting, attending religious services, being visited by a religious/spiritual leader, meditation, use of complementary and alternative therapies. Devout Muslims will pray five times a day. Some people have religious artefacts such as rosary beads, a bible or holy medals, and some people like to be visited by a member of their religious organisation.
Washing and dressing	Some Asian people may not wish to have a bath as they see the action of sitting in water as being unhygienic. Having a shower, bed bath or a bowl at the side of the bed may be a better option for them. Afro-Caribbean people may have specific skin and hair requirements which may require special oils and gels (Duffy 2008; Benson 2000). Muslim women must be kept covered, especially in the presence of men who are not in the woman's family. They are required to wear clothes that are neither transparent nor shape-revealing. Arms, legs and hair must be covered. Healthcare staff need to be aware that a Muslim woman in particular may feel uncomfortable and vulnerable being looked after in a hospital setting where she is required to wear a hospital gown or other clothing that may not meet her cultural requirements (Shamoon 2019).
Being cared for by a member of the opposite sex	Hindu, Sikh and Muslim women may have strong preferences to be treated by female care workers.

End-of-life care	Everyone will have their own idea when it comes to end-of-life care. Some will be guided by their religious, cultural or spiritual beliefs. It is important to find out by asking the client and the family.
	A Muslim may wish to sit or lie facing towards Mecca. A Sikh may receive comfort from reciting hymns from holy books (Benson 2000).
	A Buddhist may request a monk or nun be present to chant or assist the passing into the next life (Northcott 2002).
	Care following death is equally important. There may be rituals that will be required to be followed, particularly in the cleaning and handling of the body and the last offices. In order to prevent distress to family members, it would be essential that the cultural, religious and spiritual requirements of this act be established prior to the care being undertaken.

Healthcare professionals may at times have difficulty in understanding all the different types of religions and some of the traditions that go hand in hand with them. Therefore, for healthcare professionals to be competent in cultural and religious diversity, they require education and training in order to improve their knowledge and skills in handling what could be very sensitive situations. This was recognised in the HSE's National Intercultural Health Strategy 2007–2012 (HSE 2009a).

To help staff become more culturally aware and based on the recommendations of the strategy, an intercultural guide was written (HSE 2009a) identifying twenty-five communities comprising twenty-one religious groups, three ethnic/cultural groups and one group determined as 'People Without Religious Belief'. The twenty-five communities are discussed individually under seven main headings:

1. Summary of Essential Practice Points

2. Profile of the Group

3. Care of the Ill

4. Care of the Dying

5. Religious Icons and Symbols

6. Additional Notes of Maternity and Paediatric Care

7. Developing a Local Contact.

All the information provided aims to help healthcare workers develop an understanding of the various groups. The guide is extremely helpful for all healthcare workers if they are unsure about any of the listed religions or cultural groups. However, care must be exercised to avoid generalising. Each client is an individual, so it is important to use the guide as a resource and always respectfully to ask the client what their wishes are in relation to their religious and cultural needs.

Another area that we need to be mindful of is language and its potential for misinterpretation or incorrect translation. The following resources may be helpful in this regard:

HSE. (2009b). *On Speaking Terms: Good Practice Guidelines for HSE Staff in the Provision of Interpreting Services.* https://www.hse.ie/eng/services/publications/socialinclusion/emaspeaking.pdf

HSE (2012). *Lost in Translation? Good Practice Guidelines for HSE Staff in Planning, Managing and Assuring Quality Translations of Health Related Material into Other Languages.* https://www.hse.ie/eng/services/publications/ socialinclusion/lostintranslationreport.pdf

Irish Translators and Interpreters Association (ITIA) www.translatorsassociation.ie

chapter 11

PERSONAL PLANNING AND GROWTH

IN THIS CHAPTER YOU WILL LEARN ABOUT:

+ Individual goals and personal plans

+ Personal strengths and areas for development

+ Personal effectiveness

+ The concept and importance of personal planning and growth

Importance of Personal Planning and Growth

Task **Stop and think!**

What does personal planning and growth mean to you?

Spend a few minutes thinking about the areas of your life where you could develop a personal growth plan.

Personal planning and growth means thinking about ways of improving yourself so that you can become the best possible version of yourself. It is about developing self-awareness and setting long- and short-term goals. Personal growth is something that we should make every effort to do. By committing to lifelong learning and development we can hope to feel fulfilled and motivated by the goals that we set ourselves. If we don't experience personal growth, we risk becoming bored, demotivated, frustrated by lack of progress or challenge at work, and in our personal lives generally. Frankly, we could just stagnate (Robbins 2019).

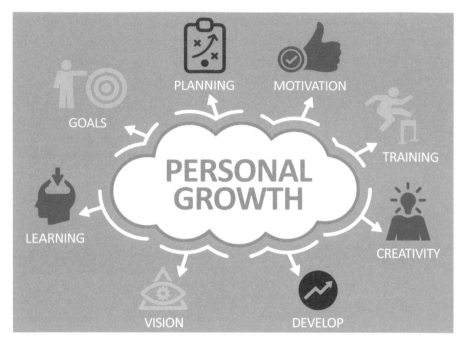

Remember, in the Hierarchy of Needs, Maslow identified that as humans we continually strive to improve ourselves and to achieve self-actualisation, the point where we reach our full potential. By undertaking the process of personal planning and growth we can set out and aim to achieve this (O'Brien 2013).

Planning involves breaking down goals into specific and achievable steps, while growth refers to personal development (Nifast 2013). We can grow physically, spiritually, emotionally, socially, intellectually and psychologically.

Personal planning and growth are important so that we can have a better sense of control over our own life. It can structure our thinking and give focus and meaning to life. It is exciting to have goals and dreams to aim towards. Planning and developing give us motivation to keep going, helping us to prioritise and maybe even change old habits that may not be healthy.

It is important to be open-minded about personal planning and growth. We need to be motivated to reach goals, aims and aspirations. Carol Dweck in her book *Mindset* (2017) talks about fixed mindsets and growth mindsets. A person with a fixed mindset believes that they can't improve themselves very much, however hard they try, therefore they consider personal planning to be of little or no value as they have closed their mind thinking, 'It won't work, so why bother; what's the point?'

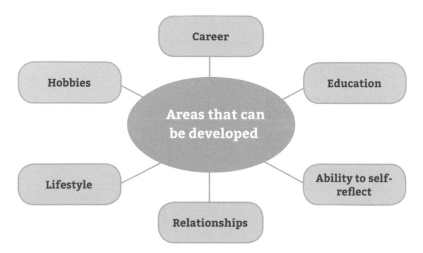

However, a person with a growth mindset takes the opposite view. They take an optimistic approach. Being open-minded, they aspire to continually improve as many aspects of their life as possible. They are prepared to set goals, plan carefully to achieve them but always ready to change their plans should the need arise or if new opportunities present themselves. They know that their hopes, plans, dreams and their full potential can be achieved through planning, training and hard work no matter how long it takes (Dweck 2017). They can overcome obstacles and setbacks through optimism and sheer hard work.

In summary: a fixed mindset generates a negative 'can't-do' attitude to personal planning and growth, whereas a growth mindset creates a positive 'can-do' attitude to personal planning and growth, and perhaps to life in general.

Personal Development Plans

Once you have decided what goals you wish to achieve and continue to develop, write down a structured personal development plan. This will help focus your mind on what you have decided to aim for, and by having something tangible such as a visual aid, you will know it's real for you. A personal development plan must be to suit you. The idea is to identify areas for further development and to set realistic, achievable, desirable goals. A personal plan helps a person to:

+ **Identify goals**: Using the SMART framework

S specific

M measurable

A attainable

R relevant

T time-based

+ **Identify reasons for the goals:** Ask yourself why you want to achieve these goals. Are they for employment? To further your career? To achieve a long-held dream?

+ **Identify ways to reach the goals:** Are there courses available? How much money would you need?

+ **Seize the moment:** Be specific about *when* you are going to work on the goals. Discipline yourself, set aside certain days of the week or times of the day to work on them. This will pay great dividends.

+ **Identify barriers:** Is it realistic to plan a full-time course if you have a full-time job? Could you instead work part-time and do the course full-time, or vice versa?

+ **Recognise help:** Who could help you – family, work colleagues, course tutors etc.?

+ **Recognise resources you may require:** Such as money, if the course is going to cost you; transport might be a problem if you don't have your own and public transport is not readily available.

+ **Monitor your progress:** Stay focused and ask for feedback from people you trust, for example, your manager, tutor or family and friends if you think they will help.

+ **Be a realistic optimist:** Reflect on past successes especially if you are having moments of self-doubt.

+ **Focus:** On what you *will do* … not on what you won't (Nifast 2013; Halverson 2011).

A personal development plan could be written in a journal or created as a vision board (Brown 2019). A vision board is a visual representation of your goals (Kane 2017).

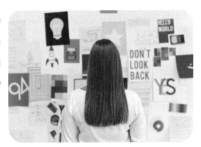

Task

Stop and think!
Using the steps above, design a personal development plan for an area of your choice e.g. career path, education, lifestyle. You can do this as a vision board, a journal or simply in your copy book.

Personal Plan Example

Area	Education
Goals (SMART)	To complete QQI Level 5 Healthcare Support Certificate
Reason for reaching the goal	To become a HCA in a nursing home
Discover how you can reach them	Attend college and hand in all assessments on time
Identify any potential barriers that may have to be overcome and consider solutions	At times I struggle with assignments and assessments
Recognise the people who may be able to help you achieve the goals	Teachers and course co-ordinators, mentor at work experience and other students

Area	Education
Resources that may be required	Notes from college, books and advice from teachers/course co-ordinators
Strengths	Attend course every day
	Communicate well with everyone
	Enjoy the course
	Hand in work on time
	Determined to succeed no matter what
Areas for development	Struggle with some modules
	Feel embarrassed to ask for help
	Nervous about work experience and not being able to do client care e.g. bed bathing
Progress/reflections (review as time goes on)	After one week of being on the course, the ups and downs
Timeframe for completion	One year (end of course)

Developing personal plans can improve personal effectiveness, meaning that we perform better as individuals, although there is always room for improvement (Nifast 2013). We can be personally effective by evaluating the goals we have set through reflective practice (see Chapter 13).

Identifying Personal Strengths and Areas for Development

We all have strengths and areas that require developing, it is part and parcel of being a human being. As a carer it is important to recognise the strengths that you require to be a carer.

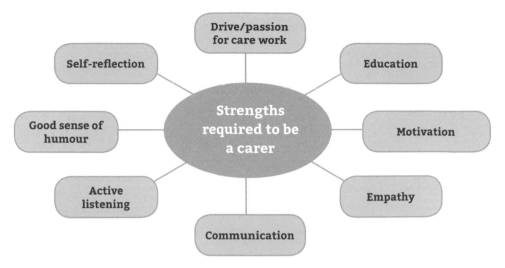

Part of personal development, planning and growth is to identify your strengths and areas for development. You can do this alone or you can ask your family and friends for help.

Identifying your strengths will give you confidence. Identifying areas for development can help with goal setting and with the construction of a meaningful development plan. For example, if you feel you talk too much (or someone tells you that you do!), then an area you may wish to develop is to practise listening more. An action plan could be to practise listening with a family member and to stay silent for longer.

Task Activity

Using the table on the next page, think about your strengths and areas for development. Using the last column, identify how you can work on the areas for development.

Use skills and experience from past work life, school life, hobbies and your own personality.

Strengths	Areas for development	Reflect on how you can develop (what action can you take?)

Personal Effectiveness

Personal effectiveness is a concept linked with wellbeing and performance. Developing personal effectiveness means examining ourselves as individuals and identifying how effective and productive we are in everyday life. This process involves self-reflection and goal setting and can be effective in the area of work or it can be done from a more holistic perspective by looking at every aspect of life e.g. relationships, interests, activities etc.

How to Be Personally Effective

Personal planning and growth is a most important starting point in developing personal effectiveness and being motivated to commence acting on the plan.

+ Be determined and have the self-confidence to achieve what you want to achieve.

+ Use reflective practice to learn about yourself and develop an understanding of different situations both in the work environment and in other areas of your life.

+ Reflect on learning in the classroom setting. This can be from the clinical skills you are learning, group discussions, making that first presentation to handing in your first assignment that you never thought you would ever complete.

+ Gain a positive attitude about yourself. Think about what you are learning and what you have learnt in the past. Look at your strengths and areas for development but see how far you have already come and what you have achieved. You may be pleasantly surprised!

+ Persistence – keep going, never give up; even if the journey takes you down a different path, keep an open mind (Dweck 2017).

+ Recognise stress and develop ways to reduce it. Taking time out, eating and sleeping well, exercising, yoga and meditation are a few things that could help.

+ Take things in small steps; you can't do everything straight away. Remember, Rome wasn't built in a day.

+ Look at how you manage time, be realistic and prioritise.

+ Journaling daily can be a useful tool to keep your head clear. Every day write down how you feel, what has happened and if you are moving forward towards your goal. You can journal in a notebook or by using a more structured format e.g. *My 90-day Morning Routine Journal* or *Happy Habits Journal* by Karen Brown.

+ Use creativity to generate new ideas, don't be afraid to explore, use vision boards so you can see you goals and plans clearly (Kane 2017).

chapter 12

PERSONAL DEVELOPMENT

IN THIS CHAPTER YOU WILL LEARN ABOUT:

+ Goals and objectives for work experience in the care environment

+ Attitudes, values and beliefs and how these may influence work practices

Goals and Objectives for Work Experience in the Care Environment

As part of the QQI requirements, learners must undertake a set amount of work experience hours during the course they are undertaking.

Prior to commencing work experience, it is important to consider the following:

+ How many hours do you need to complete in order to achieve the requirement for the course you are doing (check with the course co-ordinator or work experience tutor)?

+ How do you apply for work experience – will your college help you or do you source it yourself?

+ In which areas can you do the work experience e.g. hospital, nursing home, home care, day care centre?

+ What courses must be done prior to starting work experience e.g. patient moving and handling, infection control (handwashing), safeguarding of vulnerable people, CPR?

+ What is the dress code?

+ Will you be doing one day a week or a set block of time?

+ Will you be working shifts?

+ Do you need any paperwork such as written references, CV, photo ID?

+ Do you have the appropriate awareness of health and safety issues e.g. fire safety?

+ Will you have to do a pre-work experience interview?

Goal Setting

A good way to prepare personally prior to work experience is to identify the interpersonal, personal and practical skills that you already have. You can then identify the ones that you wish to develop during your work experience. Following work experience you can reflect on them and see if they have been developed. This is goal setting.

Task

Stop and think!
Spend a couple of minutes thinking about all the areas of your life, past employment, current employment, recent school life, hobbies, home life, voluntary work, groups you are involved in, sports you play etc.

Make a list of all the skills you can think of that you used/use in those areas, then divide them into the following categories:

+ Practical skills

+ Interpersonal skills

+ Personal skills.

Skills Audit Example

Practical	Interpersonal	Personal
Using a computer	Dealing with people	Meeting deadlines
Making things	Listening	Completing tasks
Designing things	Face-to-face interaction	Dressing professionally

Practical	Interpersonal	Personal
Using equipment	Communication skills	Being punctual
	Awareness of body language	Being patient and understanding
	Eye contact	Taking responsibility
	Being respectful	Developing knowledge
	Showing empathy	Maintaining confidentiality
	Sense of humour	

(Douglas and O'Neill 2010)

It is important to remember that all skills are transferrable and although some of the skills you are learning in the course you are undertaking may be new, you will be able to transfer old ones and develop the new ones. For example, maybe you used to work in customer services so you are used to dealing with people which is an interpersonal skill. This will be transferrable to care work as you will be dealing with clients, family members and staff in the care environment.

If you recognise your skills prior to work experience you can then set goals for work experience and identify areas you wish to develop. You can divide your goals into three sections: practical, interpersonal and personal.

Start by saying 'By the end of my work experience placement, the skills I would like to learn and develop are …'

Practical:

By the end of my work experience placement, the practical skills I would like to learn and develop are:

1. Bed bathing and bed making

2. Assisting clients with mealtimes and toileting.

Interpersonal:

By the end of my work experience placement, the interpersonal skills I would like to learn and develop are:

1. Listening and responding to clients with varying needs

2. Being aware of my body language.

Personal:

By the end of my work experience placement, the personal skills I would like to learn and develop are:

1. Using my initiative in the work environment

2. Learn more about the organisation's policies and procedures.

You may already be working as a HCA, but this exercise may be useful to you as a development tool to see what you have learnt and what areas you would like to develop. Maybe you are learning how to take blood pressure and it is a practical skill you would like to develop. If you are working, discuss your goals with your employer. If you are going on work experience, discuss them with your tutor or course co-ordinator and then your work experience mentor. Don't have too many goals as it may become unrealistic and you may feel disheartened if you don't reach those goals. Stay motivated and remember that starting something new isn't easy but you have skills that you can build on and develop.

Remember the SMART framework.

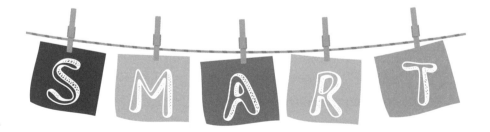

Attitudes, Values and Beliefs and How These May Influence Work Practices

As individuals we all have our own attitudes, values and beliefs towards different issues such as culture, politics, religion and ethical dilemmas e.g. abortion or punishment for crimes. Our attitudes, values and beliefs will influence how we see others including those we work with and those we care for.

Attitudes

Attitude can be seen in the ways in which we view, react or treat something or someone. As a HCA our attitude should be positive, open and warm. Our body language and facial expressions can indicate a lot so we should be mindful of this when we are with clients. Some attitudes will demonstrate a positive feeling e.g. respect, interest, patience, kindness and willingness to listen (Benson 2000).

Values

Values are our moral beliefs, principles and standards about how we should behave towards others. Values vary from person to person and culture to culture (Dustagheer et al. 2005).

As HCAs you will meet people – colleagues, clients and family members – with differing values to your own. You may find this challenging, even to the point where you feel you can't work with a certain colleague, care for a particular client or work in a certain environment.

Unaligned values may adversely influence the way you care about clients e.g. you might not spend as much time with a client whose values you don't share or you might not listen to them as well as you should. This could mean missing important information that could be critical in relation to their treatment. Likewise with colleagues who have differing values to your own, communication can become negative or abrasive, causing conflict, which in turn could easily affect the way the MDT performs. If the environment challenges your values, it could be a case of not working in that area.

As a HCA, remember that everyone has the right to be treated equally, with respect, dignity and without judgement despite their values. If you are experiencing challenges in this area, speak to the person in charge who will be able to help and guide you.

Beliefs

These are ideas and convictions that something (or things) are real or true, even if there is no evidence or proof. Beliefs can affect relationships if someone believes something to be true or real, but another person does not (Dustagheer et al. 2005).

Task **Stop and think!**
Think about your own attitudes, values and beliefs in relation to sexuality, ethnicity, culture, race, religion, politics and ethical dilemmas such as abortion. How do you feel about these topics?

Think about different groups of people in society e.g. those who have committed a crime. How would you feel about looking after them?

Prejudice, Stereotyping and Discrimination

If we let them, our beliefs, values and attitudes might well influence how we behave towards other people and they can lead to prejudice and stereotyping and discrimination.

Prejudice refers to opinions or attitudes held by members of one group towards another. It implies holding preconceived views and ideas before having any direct evidence or actual experience. We can develop prejudice through what happens in society, what we see in the media and how other people's opinions affect us. Prejudice when applied to social groups can lead to **stereotyping** about that group in the belief that everyone in that group is the same e.g. all old people are forgetful and deaf. Labelling and stereotyping can affect how people judge others and this could affect how people are cared for. An example of this could be that of a carer speaking loudly to or even shouting at older people in the belief that all old people are deaf. (Never do this – it is undignified.)

(Giddens 2001; Nolan 2003)

Circumstances where stereotyping might occur:

+ Race
+ Ethnicity
+ Sexuality
+ Nationality
+ Religious belief
+ Profession
+ Social status
+ Wealth.

Whereas prejudice is the attitude and opinion about groups and individuals, **discrimination** is the actual behaviour by someone who has prejudice towards another group or person (Giddens 2001). It is the action that leads to groups or individuals being treated badly or wrongly, from being deliberately left out or overlooked for things such as a promotion or even healthcare. It can take the form of verbal and physical abuse.

People can be discriminated against in many ways:

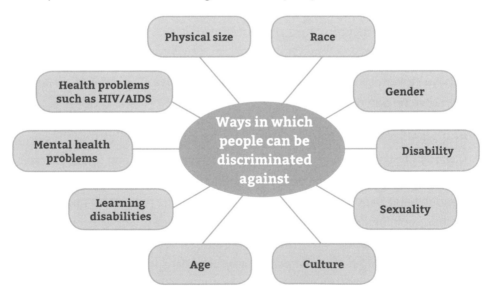

(Dustagheer et al. 2005)

Task **Stop and think!**
Can you think of any ways to prevent
discrimination, prejudice and stereotyping?

+ Cultural awareness

+ Education in schools and colleges

+ Information leaflets

+ Including everyone

+ Being non-judgemental

+ Being aware of own prejudice and stereotyping (this is not always easy as we might not think we are prejudiced)

+ Reporting any episodes of discrimination to the person in charge

+ Providing everyone with the same care to the highest possible standards.

Remember

+ Our attitudes, beliefs and values can affect the way we care about clients.

+ They can also affect the way we work within a team.

+ It is good to be aware of our attitudes, beliefs and values before we start working in healthcare.

+ If you come across a situation you have never come across before that challenges your attitudes, beliefs and values, reflect and discuss this with the person in charge.

+ Be aware of the concepts and dangers of prejudice, stereotyping and discrimination and how they are apparent in society and in healthcare. If you see any evidence in your workplace, report to the person in charge.

chapter 13
REFLECTIVE PRACTICE

IN THIS CHAPTER YOU WILL LEARN ABOUT:

✦ The concept of reflective practice   ✦ How to use reflective practice
to continuously improve one's
working methods

We do not learn from experience. We learn from reflection on experience.

(Dewey 2016)

The Concept of Reflective Practice

Reflective practice is not a new concept and has been around since the early writings of the philosopher John Dewey in 1916 (Rolfe, Freshwater and Jasper 2001). The ability to be able to reflect as a healthcare worker has become a necessary skill. Reflection is said to be a process of self–inquiry (Johns 2002). This would involve the healthcare worker developing an approach to examine themselves to learn about themselves and to develop professionally. It is about raising awareness of oneself and learning from experience. Often a difficult or uncomfortable situation (critical incident) forces us to reflect. Reflecting on both negative and positive experiences is essential so that lessons are learned and acted on in the future. Put simply, reflective practice means thinking about and analysing one's own working methods with the aim of continuous improvement for the sake of the client.

Reflection can be seen as:

A window through which the practitioner can view and focus self within the context of his/her own lived experience in ways that enable him/her confront, understand and work towards resolving the contradictions within his/her practice between what is desirable and actual practice.

(Johns 2000)

Situations We Might Reflect On

+ The death of a client

+ First day of work experience/new job

+ Conflict with client

+ Conflict with family member

+ Conflict with colleague

+ Conflict with management

+ Dealing with a client with behaviours that challenge us e.g. violence

+ A cardiac arrest

+ Helping a client who is choking

+ Helping a client following a fall

+ Admission of a new client

+ Mistakes made.

Task Stop and think!
Can you think of any other situations you could reflect on?

Many skills are required to be able to reflect critically on incidents which are concurrent with higher-order cognitive domains such as self-awareness, critical analysis, synthesis and evaluation (Burns and Bulman 2000; Rolfe, Freshwater and Jasper 2001).

Ways of Reflecting

There are two types of reflection:

1. **Reflection on-action:** Is a retrospective process whereby the practitioner reflects (or thinks) back on the positive or negative aspects of a situation to learn from what did or did not work. This can greatly assist practitioners to learn through practice and alter perceptions for past and future experiences (Atkins and Murphy 1995).

2. **Reflection in-action:** Occurs during the situation, often when there is client interaction. It involves thinking whilst acting, problem-solving and using observational skills to deal with the situation the healthcare worker is in at the time. Usually associated with more experienced practitioners. Adler puts forward that Schön sees the reflective practitioner 'as one who can think while acting and thus can respond to the uncertainty, uniqueness and conflict involved in the situations in which the professional practices' (Adler 1991; Schön 1983).

Reflection can be carried out in several different ways. You can self-reflect on your own about situations that have happened and work through them. You can debrief either formally or informally after an incident at work with a manager or co-worker. Or you can write a reflective journal, which can be your own personal journal or part of your studies. Writing reflections (or thoughts) in a journal creates a space in our busy lives. It allows us to focus on ourselves, to recognise and acknowledge who we are. You may also write reflectively in your assignments or learner records.

Reflecting on situations may trigger different and even conflicting emotions such as:

+ Guilt
+ Anger
+ Distress
+ Anxiety

+ Conflict
+ Relief
+ Happiness.

Discussing these feelings further with a colleague, manager or someone in occupational health may be a good idea or even necessary.

Reflective Frameworks

Reflective frameworks can be used by healthcare workers to assist them when undertaking reflection. They are prescriptive but can be adapted in whichever way the user may feel most beneficial in order to guide their reflection. There is a selection of frameworks available for healthcare workers to use. There are no right or wrong frameworks. The individual can decide which one works best for them. Common models include:

Gibbs' Reflective Cycle (1988)

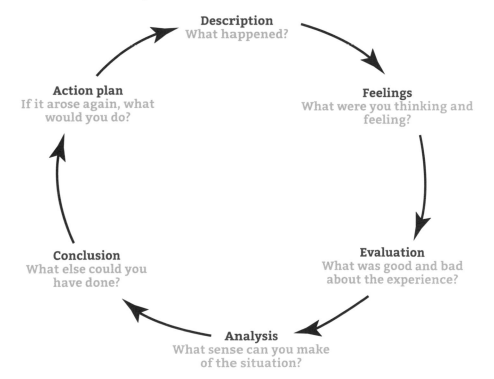

Donald Schön's Reflection On-action/Reflection In-action (1991)

Reflection in-action (at the time the event is happening)
- The experience itself
- Thinking about it during the event
- Describing how to act at the time
- Acting immediately

Reflection on-action (after the event)
- Reflecting on something that has happened
- Thinking about what you might do differently if it happened again
- New information gained and/or theoretical perspectives from study that inform the reflector's experience are used to process feeling and actions

Reflective Writing Vocabulary Aid

There are some useful prompts to consider when engaging in reflective writing:

Description – of the event/what happened	A significant event happened to me today
	The most important event that happened to me at work/work experience today
	Thinking back over the day
	Whilst reflecting on my work experience day

Feelings – what was I thinking and feeling?	I felt so surprised by my feelings of
	One of the things that surprised me was
	It was so shocking when
	I was so upset when
	I felt quite embarrassed when
	I feel happy that
	I was frustrated when
	I was positive when
Evaluation – what was good and bad about the situation?	When I think back to the situation I can see that
	Something I have found out about myself is
	I know I need to change the way I think about
	It is important for me to

Analysis – what sense can I make of the situation?	I believe that
	I still maintain that
	I understand that if I had/hadn't
	It would have been better if I had/hadn't
	I agree that
	I disagree that
Conclusion – what else could I have done?	In conclusion I can see that
	Upon reflection
	I would never have thought about the situation in this way
	The other thing I could have done was
Action plan – if it arose again what would I do?	In the future I would like to
	It is important to develop my thinking because
	Moving forward I need to
	If the situation arose again I would

(Gibbs 1988) (See also: ALIA 2013 https://www.alia.org.au/sites/default/files/ documents/Reflective%20Practice%20Vocabulary%20Aid.pdf)

Example of How to Use a Model of Reflection

Description: What Happened?	A significant event happened today in the nursing home where I work. The morning shift was busy when I was asked by another carer to help her assist one of the residents, Margaret, back to bed. Margaret was sitting in a chair. I approached her from behind and, as I bent down to greet her and make sure I was at her eye level, she grabbed me by my hair and started to shout at me. I panicked and shouted for help. Another carer quickly responded, and Margaret let go. Margaret was reassured and she calmed down and was then helped back to bed.
Feelings: What Were You Thinking and Feeling?	As I approached Margaret, I felt I was doing the right thing by cheerily greeting her and getting down to eye level. However, when she grabbed me by the hair, I was shocked – what had I done wrong? I was frightened and in pain. Margaret was very strong, and she was clearly very angry with me. I was embarrassed and felt my cheeks starting to go red. I was also anxious that I would get into trouble for causing such a stir. I was relieved when the other carer came so quickly, helping to calm Margaret down. I still felt embarrassed that it happened to me and was upset that Margaret was cross with me.
Evaluation: What Was Good and Bad about the Experience?	When I reflect on the situation, I recognised that I really admired the way that the carer responded to my cry for help and also how they managed to calm Margaret. What was bad was that I panicked and failed to react in a way that I thought I would have done before the situation arose. Recognising that I shouldn't have panicked and that I need to keep calm was positive.

Analysis: What Sense Can You Make of the Situation?	I was surprised that I panicked as I have always thought I would be very calm in this type of situation. I understand that if I hadn't approached Margaret from behind and startled her, she probably wouldn't have grabbed me by my hair. I realised that I was the trigger for her behaviour, and it was my fault that she reacted the way she did.
Conclusion	In conclusion I have realised that healthcare professionals can be the trigger for clients' behaviour. Previously challenging behaviour would have always been the fault or result of the clients' disease or disorder. I would never for a moment have thought that my actions would have caused a client to react as Margaret did that day. Reflecting on this incident taught me always to be aware that inappropriate non-verbal communication can appear to be a threat to a client.
Action Plan: If It Arose Again, What Would You Do?	If the situation arose again, I would approach the client from the front and ensure that I don't startle them. I also would remain calmer and try not to pull away from them. In the future I would like to attend a Management of Actual or Potential Aggression (MAPA) programme and, I would also like to develop my education in dementia care.

Reflect on Personal Experiences in Care Work

Task **Activity**

Using Gibbs' Reflective Cycle, reflect on any situation (positive or negative) that may have occurred in your workplace or in work experience.

Use the vocabulary aid to help you write your reflective piece.

chapter 14

ASSESSMENT GUIDELINES

The Quality and Qualifications Ireland (QQI) Level 5 Care Support Module 5N0748 is a mandatory module for the QQI Level 5 Major Healthcare Support Certificate.

QQI has two requirements that have to be met as part of the assessment process for this module. These are: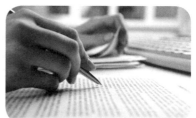

1. An assignment worth 30% of the overall mark of the module

2. A learner record worth 70% of the overall mark of the module.

Assignment 30%

Each centre will have their own assignment brief which will have been devised by the internal assessor. This brief will be designed to meet the guidelines recommended by QQI.

Students undertaking the Care Support Module are required to complete a practical activity with a client, or a group of clients, to enhance their awareness of care support in the work placement or in their work environment.

The activity must be planned, carried out and evaluated by the student and may, for example, take the form of an outing or social event for a client or group of clients. In some centres students may be able to carry out an activity where they are assisting a client with their ADLs e.g. washing and dressing a client, assisting a client with eating and drinking etc. However, this will be made clear in the assessment guidelines issued by your tutor.

The assignment may be assessed by a workplace assessor or an internal assessor working in consultation with a workplace supervisor. Evidence that this assessment took place should include a description of:

Planning the activity: The things you could consider here include

+ the activity you did

+ location of the activity

+ how you decided to do that particular activity

+ consultation and/or decision making by the client(s)

+ gaining consent from client(s) and person in charge

+ advertising/informing people about the activity

+ resources required e.g. equipment

+ who else was involved in planning the activity

+ how many people were involved

+ risk assessment/health and safety factors.

Carrying out the activity: The things you could consider here include

+ a clear description of how the activity was carried out including verbal and non-verbal communication that took place

+ the preparation of the room for the activity and the help given to the people partaking in the activity

+ details of the activity, exactly what happened, time it took place, who was involved

+ any refreshments given, any problems

+ how you completed the activity by clearing equipment away etc.

Evaluation of the activity: The things you could consider here include

+ evaluation of the impact of the activity for the client(s)

+ if you had to report anything to the person in charge

+ positive and negative outcomes

+ how you developed by doing the activity

+ what you would change

+ your strengths throughout the activity.

Task

Stop and think!

Brainstorm either on your own or with other people in your class the activities that you could do in your work placement or in your place of work. Think about the following points and make some notes that may help:

+ What resources do you have and what might you need to get if you don't have them?

+ Is it feasible for you to do the activity you would like to do?

+ Is there enough space in the location you are working in?

+ Where are you working (e.g. nursing home, hospital, intellectual disability unit, mental health services, day care centre)?

+ What is the age range of your clients?

+ Are there any health and safety issues you need to consider?

+ Can you do the activity with another member of your group (your evidence would need to be presented differently to avoid plagiarism)?

+ How much time do you have to do the activity?

+ Can you put pictures of the activity in your work?

+ How are you going to present the work (written, discussion, presentation)?

+ What are the exact guidelines you have been given by your tutor?

Examples of activities you could do for the assignment are:

✚ Bingo	✚ Reading to a client
✚ Arts and crafts	✚ Historical talk
✚ Pet therapy	✚ Poetry reading
✚ Knitting	✚ Health promotion discussion
✚ Gardening	
✚ Music afternoon	✚ Healthy eating session
✚ Pampering session	✚ Quiz
✚ Chair exercises	

✚ (other possibilities; assisting with eating and drinking, washing and dressing – check with your tutor).

Discuss your ideas with your tutor and make sure they meet the criteria for the assignment brief you have been issued and also the QQI guidelines.

You must also get permission from the person in charge in the place you are going to carry out the activity and gain consent from the clients with whom you are going to do the activity.

Learner Record 70%

As part of the QQI assessment process students are asked to complete a personal learner record. A learner record is the learner's self-reported and self-reflective record in which he/she describes specific learning experiences, activities, responses and skills acquired. This will include  reports on work carried out and interactions with others in healthcare support. This can include experience whilst on their work placement. The learner record may include:

+ reflection on relationships with clients, relatives, members of the healthcare team

+ reflection on interpersonal issues that arise in care work, such as recognising diversity and individuality in clients, families and co-workers

+ reflection on the candidate's personal effectiveness as a care worker and personal strengths and weaknesses

+ observations on the experience of receiving guidance and direction, and giving and receiving feedback

+ evidence of appropriate reporting/record-keeping

+ notes on procedures for safeguarding privacy and dignity of clients and caring for clients' property

+ notes on the structures of the health service (including personnel on the various healthcare teams).

(*Source:*https://www.qqi.ie//sites/docs/AwardsLibraryPdf/5N0758_ AwardSpecifications_English.pdf)

Each centre will have their own assignment brief which will have been devised by the internal assessor. The learner record may come in the form of a reflective diary or have structured headings. It is important to follow the guidelines set by the place you are studying in.

Task Stop and think!

On your own or with another student from your class, write down all the people you have developed a relationship with whilst on placement.

What relationship is it?

Do you have much contact with them?

Is it a good relationship and if so, in what way?

How is the communication between you?

Reflect on a particular situation when you interacted (could be a positive or negative interaction). How did it make you feel?

Task **Stop and think!**
Think about types of interpersonal issues that can arise in the workplace e.g. conflict, looking after someone from a different culture, working as part of a team or even working with a client whose behaviour challenges us. The interpersonal issue can be with anyone you have been involved with in your place of work or it may have happened in the classroom setting.

Using Gibbs' Reflective Cycle, reflect on a interpersonal issue that you have experienced.

This is an example of an extract in a learner record covering some of the points from the QQI assessment criteria. As already stated, each centre will have its own assessment brief which you must follow.

First Day of Work Experience

It was my first day of work experience in Rosevale Nursing Home. I was nervous yet excited about putting into practice the content I had learnt about in class.

During one class we had talked about our strengths and areas for development. I had written down that my strengths were that I was a good communicator, friendly and a good listener. The areas I wanted to develop were my care skills (e.g. washing and dressing clients, assisting with eating and drinking), not to be nervous around new people and develop my experiences with people with dementia. I was glad and happy we had carried out that exercise in class because I was more aware of my strengths and it gave me a little more confidence going into the work placement.

I wasn't sure which section I was going to be working in, which made me feel a little more nervous. The nursing home was a really big one with two floors and I didn't know where I was going. I tried to relax and took a deep breath as I went in. I was greeted by the Director of Nursing who told me that I would be working in 'Bluebell Unit' which was a dementia-specific unit. I was excited to be going to that unit as that was an area I want to work in and one of my personal development aims.

When I got to the unit I didn't know where to get changed or to put my bag but was met by Juliet who told me she was going to be my buddy. She seemed very friendly. Juliet showed me around and explained we would then go to the nurses station for handover. I met the team (Nurse in Charge and other HCAs) that I would be working with that day and it put me at ease to be welcomed by everyone. I also saw the doctor who was just going to see a client who had been unwell overnight. I also met the housekeeping staff who said hello and welcomed me to the nursing home.

The day started with handover when the night nurse told the day staff everything that had happened overnight with the clients, and if there had been any changes in their care. I felt really overwhelmed as I didn't know any of the clients or understand anything that anyone was talking about. I was quite lost. I think Juliet could sense that as she gave me a smile and said, 'You'll get used to it'.

Our first job was to help Bob up out of bed for a shower. Juliet and I went in to his room and she said, 'Morning Bob, we are here to give you a shower'. I was a little confused as I thought to myself, 'We are supposed to have knocked before we came into his room and we also should ask him if he wants a shower, not tell him we are going to give him one'. I didn't say anything because Juliet was being really kind to him and she has been working in the job for years. Juliet introduced me to Bob and then we helped him with a shower. A couple of times he was exposed because his towel came off and also the door to the ensuite was left open; but we quickly made sure it was shut again. We made sure the room was warm and draught-free.

Whilst we were with Bob we spoke to him about his family and how he was feeling. He was confused at times and kept asking us who we were. We reassured him the whole time we were caring for him. We kept him safe and I followed Juliet's lead and her clear direction.

Afterwards when I was tidying up I reflected on the activity I had just completed. Even though I had been taught about showering in class, it was completely different to doing it in practice. I was so glad I had Juliet with me as I don't think I would have been able to do it on my own. I didn't know what to say to Bob when he was confused and I felt a bit afraid at times in case I upset him. I didn't know where any of the equipment was and felt a bit useless at times. I have learnt to take my time, relax and take direction from my colleagues. Thank goodness Juliet was patient with me. I'm aware that it takes time to learn new skills; after all this is only day 1!

This reflective diary entry shows evidence of the following:

✚ Relationships with other healthcare workers (Juliet, nurses, doctor)

✚ Relationships with a client (Bob)

✚ Evidence of safeguarding dignity and privacy (knocking on the door, gaining consent, privacy whilst showering)

✚ Reflection on strengths and areas to develop (reflection from classroom learning and after the activity)

✚ Feelings (nervous, excited, glad, happy, confident, overwhelmed, lost, confused, afraid, useless)

✚ Reflection about the activity.

The information in this book may be a helpful aid when writing the learner record. However, a learner record is not just factual; it is a reflective piece of work which involves linking theory to practice. It is important to discuss your feelings about your experiences and what you have learnt not just in your area of work but in the classroom setting too. It is important to reflect on your strengths and the areas you need to develop and also how you are personally developing as you continue to gain experience in the areas of healthcare and education.

appendix 1

HSE'S 4 ADMINISTRATIVE AREAS AND 50 ACUTE CARE HOSPITALS

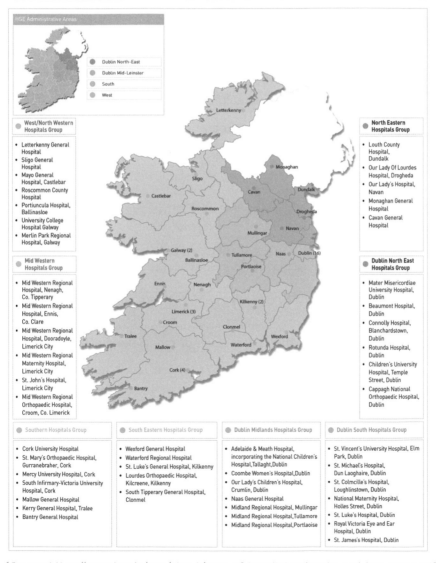

HSE Administrative Areas
- Dublin North-East
- Dublin Mid-Leinster
- South
- West

West/North Western Hospitals Group
- Letterkenny General Hospital
- Sligo General Hospital
- Mayo General Hospital, Castlebar
- Roscommon County Hospital
- Portiuncula Hospital, Ballinasloe
- University College Hospital Galway
- Merlin Park Regional Hospital, Galway

Mid Western Hospitals Group
- Mid Western Regional Hospital, Nenagh, Co. Tipperary
- Mid Western Regional Hospital, Ennis, Co. Clare
- Mid Western Regional Hospital, Dooradoyle, Limerick City
- Mid Western Regional Maternity Hospital, Limerick City
- St. John's Hospital, Limerick City
- Mid Western Regional Orthopaedic Hospital, Croom, Co. Limerick

North Eastern Hospitals Group
- Louth County Hospital, Dundalk
- Our Lady Of Lourdes Hospital, Drogheda
- Our Lady's Hospital, Navan
- Monaghan General Hospital
- Cavan General Hospital

Dublin North East Hospitals Group
- Mater Misericordiae University Hospital, Dublin
- Beaumont Hospital, Dublin
- Connolly Hospital, Blanchardstown, Dublin
- Rotunda Hospital, Dublin
- Children's University Hospital, Temple Street, Dublin
- Cappagh National Orthopaedic Hospital, Dublin

Southern Hospitals Group
- Cork University Hospital
- St. Mary's Orthopaedic Hospital, Gurranebraher, Cork
- Mercy University Hospital, Cork
- South Infirmary-Victoria University Hospital, Cork
- Mallow General Hospital
- Kerry General Hospital, Tralee
- Bantry General Hospital

South Eastern Hospitals Group
- Wexford General Hospital
- Waterford Regional Hospital
- St. Luke's General Hospital, Kilkenny
- Lourdes Orthopaedic Hospital, Kilcreene, Kilkenny
- South Tipperary General Hospital, Clonmel

Dublin Midlands Hospitals Group
- Adelaide & Meath Hospital, incorporating the National Children's Hospital, Tallaght, Dublin
- Coombe Women's Hospital, Dublin
- Our Lady's Children's Hospital, Crumlin, Dublin
- Naas General Hospital
- Midland Regional Hospital, Mullingar
- Midland Regional Hospital, Tullamore
- Midland Regional Hospital, Portlaoise

Dublin South Hospitals Group
- St. Vincent's University Hospital, Elm Park, Dublin
- St. Michael's Hospital, Dun Laoghaire, Dublin
- St. Colmcille's Hospital, Loughlinstown, Dublin
- National Maternity Hospital, Holles Street, Dublin
- St. Luke's Hospital, Dublin
- Royal Victoria Eye and Ear Hospital, Dublin
- St. James's Hospital, Dublin

(*Source*: https://www.hse.ie/eng/about/map-of-hospital-networks-and-hse-areas.pdf)

SLÁINTECARE

Sláintecare – A Pathway to Universal Healthcare in Ireland

What Is Sláintecare?

Sláintecare is a vision for a new health service in Ireland detailed in the report from the Oireachtas Committee on the Future of Healthcare published on 30 May 2017.

It is the first time there has been political consensus on a health reform plan for the next ten years and cross-party support on delivering a universal health system in Ireland.

What Are the Main Components of Sláintecare?

Sláintecare will provide:

+ Entitlement for all Irish residents to all health and social care

+ No charge to access GP, primary or hospital care and reduced charges for drugs

+ Care provided at the lowest level of complexity, often outside of hospital, in an integrated way

+ eHealth as key tool for developing a universal health system and integrated care

+ Strong focus on public health and health promotion

+ Waiting times guarantees with a maximum:

  - 4-hour wait time for Emergency Departments

  - 10 days for a diagnostics test

- − 10 weeks for an out-patient appointment
- − 12 weeks for an in-patient procedure
- ✛ Private care phased out of public hospitals
- ✛ Significant expansion of access to diagnostics in the community
- ✛ Earlier and better access to mental health services
- ✛ An expanded workforce including allied health professionals, nurses and doctors. The importance of addressing recruitment and retention issues of all healthcare staff and the development of integrated workforce planning is emphasised in the report.
- ✛ A new HSE Board, to be established promptly
- ✛ Accountability and clinical governance, to be legislated for
- ✛ A National Health Fund set up to ring-fence funding for a transitional fund and expansion of entitlements.

The report sets out specific costings for the expansion of entitlements and system development and timelines for implementation, recommending the establishment of an Implementation Office to drive the reform.

How Long Will It Take to Do This?

The report is for a ten-year period but many of the key actions will be implemented during the first six years.

How Much Will It Cost?

The expansion of entitlements detailed in the report will cost an additional €2.8 billion by year ten, with a one-off transitional fund of €3 billion required over the first six years for infrastructure investment, expansion of training capacity and the timely implementation of the eHealth strategy.

(*Source*: Centre for Health Policy and Management, TCD; HRB funded Pathways to Universal Healthcare Project)

(For further reading: https://www.gov.ie/en/campaigns/slaintecare-implementation-strategy/)

NATIONAL JOB DESCRIPTION FOR THE HCA

Job Description for Health Care Assistant (HCA)

Introduction

The role of the HCA is to support the delivery of patient care under the supervision and direction of qualified nursing personnel (Shannon et al. 2001). Nursing has been defined as 'The use of clinical judgement in the provision of care to enable people to improve, maintain, or recover health, to cope with health problems, and to achieve the best quality of life, whatever their disease or disability, until death' (Royal College of Nursing 2003).

The difference between the registered nurse and the HCA is in the knowledge that is the basis of the assessment of need and the determination of action to meet the need, plus the clinical judgement inherent in the processes of assessment, diagnosis, prescription and evaluation.

Educational Qualifications

The recognised qualification for HCAs is the QQI Level 5 Healthcare Support Certificate. Staff engaged in the role of HCA but who have not yet completed this programme can continue in their role and the agreed job description will apply to them. These and all newly recruited HCAs will be required to undertake the qualification as soon as it can be available to them.

In exceptional circumstances individual staff members may not be able to undertake and complete the training for the qualification. In this context the job description should consider that the HCA has not been trained in all aspects covered by the qualification. In other words, a HCA who has not taken the qualification should not be expected to take on the range of duties that a qualified HCA could undertake.

Title

The title Health Care Assistant (HCA) should be used nationally.

Responsibility

There is a clear report relationship between the HCA and the clinical nurse manager or their deputy.

Accountability

HCAs are accountable for their actions in the delivery of patient care and must not undertake any duty related to patient care for which he/she is not trained, in accordance with the educational qualifications outlined above.

The HCA must report to and work under the supervision and direction of a registered nurse in relation to their duties/tasks and must be integrated into the ward/area team.

Nursing staff will delegate duties in accordance with their professional judgement and within the competence, that is the training, knowledge and experience of the HCA.

Nursing staff must not allocate any duty to the HCA for which he/she has not been trained.

16 Key Activities

There are 16 key activities where patients/clients may require assistance as part of daily living.

The duty of the registered nurse is to assess, plan, implement and evaluate the care required by the patient. The primary role of the HCA is to assist the nurse in the implementation of that care, as determined by the registered nurse. Duties assigned to the HCA will vary depending on the care setting and will include the following functions. This is not an exhaustive list.

+ To carry out assigned and delegated tasks involving direct care and all Activities of Daily Living (ADLs) under the supervision of a registered nurse (e.g. to assist clients maintain standards of personal hygiene, laundry, dietary intake, physical and mental health).

+ Assisting the registered nurse in the provision of quality nursing service by promoting and adopting a philosophy of care within the service area.

+ Assisting the registered nurse in duties associated with the delivery of care and management of the ward/healthcare environment and other support duties as appropriate.

+ To report any incident or potential incident which may compromise the health and safety of clients, staff or visitors and take whatever appropriate action they can.

+ HCAs should always conduct themselves in a manner that shows respect for the individual and ensures safe patient care.

So, to emphasise, the personal characteristics that indicate these principles should include:

+ Confidentiality
+ Communication
+ Courtesy
+ Dignity and privacy
+ Accountability
+ Health and safety.

REFERENCES

Adler, S. (1991). 'The reflective practitioner and the curriculum of teacher education'. *Journal of Education for Teaching.* 17/2, 39–149.

Aihong, R. (2014). '"Who am I": Alice's quest for knowledge and identity in Wonderland'. *Studies in Literature and Language.* 8/3, 126–132.

Angelou, M. (2014). *Rainbow in the Cloud: The Wisdom and Spirit of Maya Angelou.* Random House.

Allen, R. (ed). (2001). *The Penguin Concise English Dictionary.* London: Penguin Group.

Amy Speech and Language Therapy Inc. (2010). 'Augmentative and alternative communication devices (AAC)'. <https://www.amyspeechlanguagetherapy.com/communication-boards.html>

Anderson, K.N., Anderson, L.E. and Glanze, W.D. (1994). *Mosby's Medical, Nursing and Allied Health Dictionary* (4th edn). St Louis: Mosby Year Book, Inc.

Atkins, S. and Murphy, K. (1995). 'Reflective practice'. *Nursing Standard.* 9/45, 31–37.

Australian Library and Information Association (ALIA). (2013). 'Reflective practice writing guide: A guide to getting started'. <http://www.alia.org.au/sites/default/files/documents/Reflective.Practice.Writing.Guide20130409JB.pdf>

Beach, M.C., Duggan, P.S., Cassel, C.K. and Gellar, G. (2007). 'What does "respect" mean? Exploring the moral obligation of health professionals to respect patients'. *Journal of General Internal Medicine.* 22/5, 692–695.

Beauchamp, T.L. and Childress, J.F. (2013). *Principles of Biomedical Ethics* (7th edn). Oxford: Oxford University Press. Cited in Elcock, K., Wright, W., Newcombe, P. and Everett, F. (eds). (2019). *Essentials of Nursing Adults.* London: SAGE Publications Ltd.

Belbin. 'The nine Belbin team roles'. <https://www.belbin.com/about/belbin-team-roles/>

Benson, S. (ed). (2000). *Handbook for Care Assistants: A Practical Guide to Caring for Elderly People* (5th edn). London: Hawker Publications Ltd.

British Columbia Rehabilitation Society (BCRS), now Vancouver Hospital and Health Science Centre (VHHSC). (1992). National Council of State Boards of Nursing (NCSBN). (2018). *A Nurse's Guide to Professional Boundaries.* Chicago: NCSBN. <https://www.ncsbn.org/ProfessionalBoundaries_Complete.pdf>

Brown, K. (2019). *Happy Habits Journal.* Wrocklam: Amazon Fulfillment.

---- *My 90-Day Morning Routine Journal.* Wrocklam: Amazon Fulfillment.

Burns, S. and Bulman, C. (eds). (2000). *Reflective Practice in Nursing – The Growth of the Professional Practitioner* (2nd edn). Oxford: Blackwell Science Ltd.

CARNA - College and Association of Registered Nurses of Alberta (CARNA) (2011) Professional Boundaries for Registered Nurses Guidelines for the Nurse-Client Relationship. Available online: https://www.nurses.ab.ca/docs/default-source/document-library/guidelines/rn_professional-boundaries.pdf?sfvrsn=cc43bb24_14

Carter, P.J. and Goldschmidt, W.M. (2010). *Lippincott's Textbook for Long-Term Care Nursing Assistants: A Humanistic Approach to Caregiving.* Philadelphia: Wolters Kluwer/Lippincott Williams and Wilkins.

Central Statistics Office. (2019). Census 2016 Reports. <https://www.cso.ie/en/census/census2016reports/>

Centre for Health Policy and Management. (2019). 'Sláintecare – A Pathway to Universal Healthcare in Ireland'. Dublin: Trinity College Dublin. <https://www.tcd.ie/medicine/health_policy_management/assets/pdf/policy-brief-on-the-slaintecare-report-19122017.pdf>

Citizens Information (2019) Charges for Hospital Services. Available online. https://www.citizensinformation.ie/en/health/health_services/gp_and_hospital_services/hospital_charges.html

---- Citizens Information. 'Employee's rights and entitlements'. <https://www.citizensinformation.ie/en/employment/employment_rights_and_conditions/employment_rights_and_duties/employee_rights_and_entitlements.html>

College of Nurses of Ontario (CNO). (2006) *Practice Standard: Therapeutic Nurse–Client Relationship, Revised 2001.* Toronto: CNO. <https://www.cno.org/en/learn-about-standards-guidelines/educational-tools/learning-modules/therapeutic-nurse-client-relationship/>

Dahlgren and Whitehead. (1992). 'The determinants of health'. In Elcock, K., Wright, W., Newcombe, P. and Everett, F. (eds). (2019). *Essentials of Nursing Adults.* London: SAGE Publications Ltd.

Department of Health (DOH). (1994). *Shaping a Healthier Future: A Strategy for Effective Health Care in the 1990s.* Dublin: Government Publications ISBN: 0-70760374-9.

---- (1998). *Report on the Commission on Nursing, A Blueprint for the Future.* Dublin: Government Publications. <https://health.gov.ie/blog/publications/report-of-the-commission-on-nursing/>

---- (2000). *National Health Promotion Strategy 2000–2005.* Dublin: Government Publications.

---- (2001). *Primary Care A New Direction Quality and Fairness – A Health System for You.* Dublin: Government Publications ISBN 0-7557-1179-3. <https://health.gov.ie/wp-content/uploads/2014/03/primcare-report.pdf>

---- (2001a). *Quality and Fairness: A Health System for You.* Dublin: Government Publications.

---- (2001b). *Primary Care: A New Direction for You.* Dublin: Government Publications. <https://health.gov.ie/wp-content/uploads/2014/03/primcare-report.pdf>

---- (2011). *Effective Utilisation of Professional Skills of Nurses and Midwives Report of the Working Group.* <https://health.gov.ie/wp-content/uploads/2014/03/Effective-Utilisation-of-Professional-Skills-of-Nurses-and-Midwives-Report.pdf>

---- (2013). *Health Ireland: A Framework for Improved Health and Wellbeing 2013–2025.* <https://health.gov.ie/wp-content/uploads/2014/03/HealthyIrelandBrochureWA2.pdf>

Department of Transport, Tourism and Sport (DDTAS), Department of Health (DOH). (2013). *Healthy Ireland: A Framework for Improved Health and Wellbeing 2013–2016.* Dublin: Government Publications.

Dewey, J. (1916). *Democracy and Education.* New York: Macmillan.

Dignity in Care Campaign. <https://www.dignityincare.org.uk/About/Dignity_in_Care_campaign/>

Douglas, A. and O'Neill, S. (2010). *The Essential Work Experience Handbook* (3rd edn). Dublin: Gill and Macmillan.

Duffy, I. (2008). *Healthcare Support: A Textbook for Healthcare Assistants.* Dublin: Gill and Macmillan.

Dustagheer, A., Harding, J. and McMahon, C. (2005). *Knowledge to Care: A Handbook for Care Assistants* (2nd edn). Oxford: Blackwell Publishing.

Dweck, C. (2017). *Mindset.* London: Robinson.

Elcock, K., Wright, W., Newcombe, P., Everett, F. (eds). (2019). *Essentials of Nursing Adults.* London: SAGE Publications Ltd.

Everyday Health. (2017). '7 Guidelines for accepting constructive criticism'. <https://www.everydayhealth.com/healthy-living/7-guidelines-accepting-constructive-criticism/>

Fleming, I. (2004). *Teamworking Pocketbook* (2nd edn). Hants: Management Pocketbooks Ltd.

Geary, L.M. (2004). *Medicine and Charity in Ireland 1718–1851.* Dublin: UCD Press.

Geary, L.M., Lynch, B. and Turner, B. (2018). *The Irish Healthcare System, A Historical and Comparative Review.* Dublin: Dublin Health Insurance Authority (HIA). <https://www.hia.ie/sites/default/files/The%20Irish%20Healthcare%20System%20-%20An%20Historical%20and%20Comparative%20Review_0.pdf>

Gibbs, G. (1988). *Learning by Doing: A Guide to Teaching and Learning Methods.* London: Further Education Unit.

Giddens, A. (2001). *Sociology* (4th edn). Cambridge: Polity Press.

Goodwin Chew, H. (2011). 'Ethics and spirituality in care'. In *Concepts of Care: A Text Book for Health Care Assistants.* Kerry: Leading Healthcare Providers (LHP) Skillnet.

Greene, C. (2011). 'Essential preparation for the health care assistants caring role.' In *Concepts of Care: A Text Book for Health Care Assistants.* Kerry: Leading Healthcare Providers (LHP) Skillnet.

Halverson, H.G. (2011). *9 Things Successful People Do Differently.* Boston: Harvard Business Review Press.

Hardavella, G., Aamali-Gaagnat, A., Saad, N. et al. (2017). 'How to give and receive feedback effectively'. *Breathe.* 13/4, 327–333. <https://www.ncbi.nlm.nih.gov/pmc/articles/PMC5709796/>

Health Information and Quality Authority (HIQA). (2016). *National Standards for Residential Care Settings for Older People in Ireland.* <https://www.hiqa.ie/sites/default/files/2017-01/National-Standards-for-Older-People.pdf>

Health Service Executive (HSE). (2006). *Report of the High Level Group on Health Care Assistants Regarding the Implementation of the Health Care Assistants.* <https://www.hse.ie/eng/staff/resources/hrstrategiesreports/report%20of%20the%20high%20level%20group%20on%20health%20care%20assistants%20regarding%20the%20implementation%20of%20the%20hca%20programme.pdf>

---- (2009a). *Health Services Intercultural Health Guide Responding to the Needs of Diverse Religious Communities and Cultures in Healthcare Settings.* <https://www.hse.ie/eng/services/publications/socialinclusion/interculturalguide/>

---- (2009b) *On Speaking Terms: Good Practice Guidelines for HSE Staff in the Provision of Interpreting Services.* <https://www.hse.ie/eng/services/publications/socialinclusion/emaspeaking.pdf>

---- (2012) *Lost in Translation? Good Practice Guidelines for HSE Staff in Planning, Managing and Assuring Quality Translations of Health Related Material into Other Languages.* <https://www.hse.ie/eng/services/publications/socialinclusion/lostintranslationreport.pdf>

---- (2011).*The Health Promotion Strategic Framework.* <https://www.healthpromotion.ie/hp-files/docs/HPSF_HSE.pdf>

---- (2012). *National Dementia Education Programme.* <https://www.hse.ie/eng/services/publications/nursingmidwifery%20services/dementia.html>

---- (2014). *Safeguarding Vulnerable Persons at Risk of Abuse National Policy and Procedures. Incorporating Services for Elder Abuse and Persons with a Disability Social Care Division.* <https://www.hse.ie/eng/services/publications/corporate/personsatriskofabuse.pdf>

---- (2015). *Building a High Quality Health Service for a Healthier Ireland Health Service Executive Corporate Plan 2015–2017.* <https://www.hse.ie/eng/services/publications/corporate/corporateplan15-17.pdf>

---- (2018) Our Structure. Available online: https://www.hse.ie/eng/about/who/

---- (2018) Hospital Charges. Available online. https://www.hse.ie/eng/about/who/acute-hospitals-division/patient-care/hospital-charges/

---- (2018a). 'About Primary Care Teams (PCTs)'. <https://www.hse.ie/eng/services/list/2/primarycare/pcteams/>

---- (2018b). *Second National Intercultural Health Strategy 2018–2023.* <https://www.hse.ie/eng/about/who/primarycare/socialinclusion/intercultural-health/intercultural-health-strategy.pdf>

'HSELanD available for HSE employees'. <https://www.hseland.ie/dash/Account/Login>

Heartsaver CPR (now Irish Heart Foundation). (2019). 'Courses for healthcare professionals'. <https://irishheart.ie/your-health/cpr/healthcare-professionals/>

'Hello my name is campaign'.<https://www.hellomynameis.org.uk/>

Hensey, B. (1988). *The Health Services of Ireland* (4th edn). Dublin: Institute of Public Administration.

Hindle, A. and Coates, A. (eds). (2011). *Nursing Care of Older People: A Textbook for Students and Nurses.* Oxford: Oxford University Press.

Irish Hospice Foundation (IHF) (2013). *Module 7: The Ethics of Keeping Confidentiality.* <http://hospicefoundation.ie/wp-content/uploads/2013/10/Module-7-The-Ethics-of-Confidentiality-and-Privacy.pdf>

(IHF) 'Design and dignity programme'. <https://hospicefoundation.ie/design-dignity/>

Irish Translators and Interpreters Association (ITIA) <www.translatorsassociation.ie>

Jay, R. (2003). *How to Build a Great Team.* Harlow: Pearson Education Limited.

Johns, C. (1995). 'Framing learning through reflection within Carper's fundamental ways of knowing in nursing'. *Journal of Advanced Nursing.* 22, 226–234.

---- (2000). *Becoming a Reflective Practitioner.* Oxford: Blackwell Science Ltd.

---- (2002). *Guided Reflection Advancing Practice.* Oxford: Blackwell Science Ltd.

Kane, C. (2017). *The Complete Guide to Vision Boards.* Christine Kane.

LGBT Ireland (2018) About Sexuality and Romantic Identities. Available online: https://lgbt.ie/get-information/sexuality-and-romantic-identities/

Mahoney, F.I. and Barthel, D.W. (1965). 'Functional evaluation: The Barthel index'. *Maryland State Medical Journal.* 14, 61–65.

Mairis, E.D. (1994). 'Concept clarification in professional practice – dignity'. *Journal of Advanced Nursing.* 19, 947–953.

McCorry, L.K. and Mason, J. (2011). *Communication Skills for the Healthcare Professional.* Baltimore: Lippincott Williams and Wilkins.

McGinn, P. 'Legal dialogue: Confidentiality issues'. <https://www.inmo.ie/Article/PrintArticle/1034>

Milgram, J. (1992) Boundaries in professional relationship: a training manual. Minneapolis, Minnesota: Walk-In Counselling Centre. Cited in British Columbia College of Nursing Professionals (2019) Professional versus personal relationships. Available online: https://www.bccnp.ca/Standards/all_nurses/resources/boundaries/Pages/PersonalVProfessional.aspx

Mitchell, G., Cousins, C., Burrows, T. and Cousins, G. (2017). 'A review of safe-staffing models and their applicability to care homes'. *Journal of Nursing Management.* 25/2, 157–162. <https://doi.org/10.1111/jonm.12450>

National Council of State Boards of Nursing (NCSBN). (2018). *A Nurse's Guide to Professional Boundaries.* Chicago, IL: NCSBN. <https://www.ncsbn.org/ProfessionalBoundaries_Complete.pdf>

Nazarko, L. (2000). *NVQs in Nursing and Residential Care Homes* (2nd edn). Oxford: Blackwell Science Ltd.

Nelson-Jones, R. (2004). *Effective Thinking Skills.* London: Sage Publications Ltd.

Nifast. (2013). *Care of the Older Person FETAC Level 5.* Dublin: Gill and Macmillan.

Nifast. (2013). *Care Skills and Care Support FETAC Level 5.* Dublin: Gill and Macmillan.

Nightingale, F. (1859, 1992, p.70) citied in Irish Hospice Foundation, Hospice Friendly Hospitals Module 7 The Ethics of Keeping Confidentiality. Available online: http://hospicefoundation.ie/wp-content/uploads/2013/10/Module-7-The-Ethics-of-Confidentiality-and-Privacy.pdf

Nolan, Y. (2003.) *Care* (2nd edn). Oxford: Heinemann Educational Publishers.

Northcott, N. (2002). 'Nursing with dignity part 2: Buddhism'. *Nursing Times.* 98/10, 36–38.

Nova Scotia College of Nursing. (NSCN). (2019). Professional boundaries and the nurse–client relationship. <https://cdn1.nscn.ca/sites/default/files/documents/resources/ProfessionalBoundaries.pdf>

Nursing and Midwifery Board of Ireland (NMBI). (2014). *Code of Professional Conduct and Ethics for Registered Nurses and Registered Midwives.* Dublin: NMBI. <https://www.nmbi.ie/NMBI/media/NMBI/Code-of-professional-Conduct-and-EthicsAd_2.pdf?ext=.pdf>

O'Brien, E.Z. (2013). *Human Growth and Development: An Irish Perspective* (2nd edn). Dublin: Gill and Macmillan.

O'Dowd, A. (2009). 'HCAs and patient confidentiality'. <https://www.nursingtimes.net/hcas-and-patient-confidentiality/5000408.article>

Oram, H. (2009). 'An Irishman's Diary'. Dublin: *Irish Times.* <https://www.irishtimes.com/opinion/an-irishman-s-diary-1.744747>

Parkinson's UK. 'Speech and communication problems in Parkinson's'. <https://www.parkinsons.org.uk/information-and-support/speech-and-communication-problems-parkinsons>

Parkinsons UK (No Date). https://www.parkinsons.org.uk/information-and-support/speech-and-communication-problems-parkinsons accessed 20/6/2019

Power, G. (2019). *Complete Care Skills.* Tipperary: Boru Press Ltd.

Power, M. and Duffy, I. (eds). *Concepts of Care: A Text Book for Health Care Assistants.* Kerry: Leading Healthcare Providers (LHP) Skillnet.

Rolfe, G., Freshwater, D. and Jasper, M. (2001). *Critical Reflection for Nursing and the Helping Professions – A User's Guide.* Palgrave: Hampshire.

Roper, N., Logan, W.W. and Tierney, A.J. (1996). *The Elements of Nursing: A Model for Nursing Based on a Model of Living* (4th Edition). Edinburgh: Churchill Livingstone.

---- (2000). *The Roper-Logan-Tierney Model of Nursing: Based on Activities of Living.* Edinburgh: Elsevier Health Sciences.

Robbins, T. 'How to create a personal growth plan'. <https://www.tonyrobbins.com/productivity-performance/how-to-create-personal-growth-plan/>

Rootman I. (2001). 'A framework for health promotion evaluation'. The National Centre for Biotechnology Information (NCBI). PubMed. <https://www.ncbi.nlm.nih.gov/pubmed/11729789>

Royal College of Nursing (RCN). (2003). 'Defining nursing'. <http://www.rcn.org.uk/downloads/definingnursing/definingnursing-a5.pdf>

---- (2016). 'What person-centred care means'. <https://rcni.com/hosted-content/rcn/first-steps/what-person-centred-care-means>

Schempp, D. (2014). 'Emotional side of caregiving'. Family Caregiver Alliance (FCA).<https://www.caregiver.org/emotional-side-caregiving>

Schön, D.A. (1991). *The Reflective Turn: Case Studies In and On Educational Practice.* New York: Teachers Press, Columbia University.

Shamoon, Z. (2019). 'Cultural competence in the care of the Muslim patient and their families'. <https://www.ncbi.nlm.nih.gov/pubmed/29763108>

Stroke Association. (2012). 'Communication problems after stroke'. <https://www.stroke.org.uk/sites/default/files/Communication%20problems%20after%20stroke.pdf >

Stroke Association Information Service (2012). https://www.stroke.org.uk/sites/default/files/Communication%20probems%20after%20stroke.pdf

World Health Organization (WHO). (1986). Ottowa Charter for Health Promotion. First International conference on health promotion 17–21 November, Ottowa. Copenhagen: WHO Regional Office for Europe.

University Hospitals Birmingham (UHB). (2019). NHS Foundation Trust. 'Privacy and dignity'. <https://www.uhb.nhs.uk/privacy-and-dignity.htm>

USEFUL WEBSITES

Active Minds: *www.active-minds.org/uk*

Active Retirement Ireland: *www.activeirl.ie*

Age Action: *www.ageaction.ie*

Age and Opportunity: *www.ageandopportunity.ie*

Alzheimer Society of Ireland: *www.alzheimer.ie*

Communication Matters: *www.communicationmatters.org.uk*

Dementia Care Matters: *www.dementiacarematters.com*

Dementia Understand Together: *www.understandtogether.ie*

Health and Safety Authority (HAS): *www.hsa.ie*

Health Information and Quality Authority (HIQA): *www.hiqa.ie*

Health Service Executive (HSE): *www.hse.ie*

Irish Heart Foundation: *www.irishheart.ie*

Irish Hospice Foundation: *www.hospicefoundation.ie*

Parkinson's Association of Ireland: *www.parkinsons.ie*

Stroke Association: *www.stroke.org.uk*

World Health Organisation: *www.who.int*

INDEX